The Road Back Program

How to Get Off

Psychoactive
Drugs
Safely

There is Hope.

There is a Solution.

By James Harper
with Jayson Austin

DISCLAIMER

The claims, information and products mentioned in this book, The Road Back Program, How to Get Off Psychoactive Drugs Safely, have not been evaluated by the United States Food and Drug Administration and are not approved to diagnose, treat, cure or prevent disease.

The information provided in the book, The Road Back Program How to Get Off Psychoactive Drugs Safely, is for informational purposes only and is not intended as a substitute for advice from your physician or other health- care professional.

You should not use the information in this book for diagnosis or treatment of any health problem or for prescription of any medication or other treatment.

You should consult with a health-care professional before starting any diet, exercise or supplementation program, before taking any medication, or if you have, or suspect that you might have a health problem.

CONTENTS

INTRODUCTION

BY JAMES HARPER

AFTER FOURTEEN YEARS of research, assisting tens of thousands of people to get off their psychoactive medication, this book is the final and closing chapter of the development of The Road Back Program. Not to say there will not be future advancements in this program, but the needed foundation for a psychoactive withdrawal program and health program is now firmly in place. The success rate of people now using this program is higher than ever imagined, the basic causes of drug withdrawal symptoms and the human health decline have now been discovered, and the solution is backed by scientific evidence.

This book is written mainly for the patient, or individual wanting to get off their drug or to simply rebuild or maintain good health. The last chapter of this book details the science behind this program and is written for the health-care provider.

If you have tried to get off your medication in the past and suffered, have found this book in the middle of your withdrawal or quit the drug cold turkey, you may have a little more work to do than most, but the success will still be there. With the advancements in The Road Back Program your route to recovery and feeling well again or maybe feeling well for the first time in years can now be accomplished in a rather short amount of time.

If you are seeking to improve your overall health, there is usually no need to be patient when you use the program, it works rather quickly. Many of us are just accustomed to feeling how we feel and we may have lost track of how good we can feel when the body and mind work as a unique team. By doing a few basic things, we can reverse much of what is happening inside of our body and that reversal usually equates to a better attitude in life and a major quality of life improvement.

I want to acknowledge the many of people, from the four corners of Earth and all walks of life, who have successfully changed their life while using this program. Their perseverance and feedback have helped advance this program to today's high degree of success.

And I applaud you, opening this book for the first time, for your courage and resolve to change your life and get yourself back as your reward.

I understand the apprehension you may feel about deciding to come off the drug, especially if you have tried to do so before and failed, or if you have heard horror stories of others who have tried to come off psychoactive medication.

Further, I understand the questions you might be asking at this point:

• *Will I experience mental or physical pain while on this program?*

• *Will I have other side effects while on this program?*

• *Will the drug side effects get worse before they get better?*

• *Will my depression get worse during this program?*

• *Will my anxiety levels increase?*

You may have many other questions in addition to those above, but most importantly you should know that The Road Back Program is virtually side effect free. The testament to this, as you will see throughout the book, is that people just like you start to feel better, mentally and physically, sometimes from day one.

The program is set-up so that you usually only start reducing the drug after you feel a major positive change and all or nearly all-existing side effects from the drug are eliminated. Thus, you know from the very beginning, change is possible; that this time there is a chance for you, and that you can do this and feel well once again.

The program is simple, effective, and extremely powerful: when applied correctly. You too can have resounding success in getting off the medication and getting your life back.

Based on extensive research, specific "nutrients" have been formulated for this program. Their use, in conjunction with the full and complete program, have resulted in a high success rate of people getting off psychoactive medication, while also enormously reducing the potential and feared side effects from withdrawal.

What unwanted feelings come from you and what feelings does the medication generate? The program separates these confusing symptoms, and once this separation occurs, the real you will emerge.

One major change most people experience during the program; their reach for life returns or truly begins for the first time. Reach is defined as: to extend out; to touch or to seize; to communicate with.

Life is defined as: the quality that distinguishes a *vital* and functional being from a dead body or inanimate matter (Webster's Dictionary). Per the definition of life, *you* are vital. We need you and humankind needs you. The positive changes you can bring to others are beyond imagining. Life can be grand, life can be fulfilling; you, changing your life and having "reach" return will absolutely affect others in your environment.

Reach can return with your children, spouse, work or activities you have been putting off for years that you have always wanted to do, or to do once again.

Remember and hold the following close to your heart as you travel this journey:

• You Can Change.

• You Can Change How You Feel.

• You Can Be a Positive Influence for Others.

• You Can Make It.

Antidepressants are often prescribed for post-menopausal symptoms without full knowledge of the risk/benefit equation. During 2009, two studies were published that still stick in my mind and need sharing.

It is acknowledged by the medical community that there is an increased risk for heart disease and stroke for post-menopausal women taking antidepressants. Antidepressants do work somewhat like aspirin, helps thin the blood, helps stop clotting, and with a few percentage points above a placebo in clinical trials, will work for depression or anxiety.

That is the benefit of antidepressants. What are the risk factors?

In December 2009, a troubling antidepressant study was published in Archives of Internal Medicine.

136,000 women participants enrolled in the Women's Health Initiative study. None were taking an antidepressant at the time of enrollment.

- The women had their first follow-up visit between year 1 and year 3.

- During their follow-up visit, 5,500 women had started taking an antidepressant.

- The researchers found that the women taking an antidepressant had a 45% increase in the risk of stroke.

- There was a 32% increase risk of dying from any cause during the follow-up period with the women taking an antidepressant.

- The older tricyclic antidepressants were not linked to stroke, but they did increase the risk of dying by 67% during follow-up. Jordan W. Smoller, M.D., ScD, of the Massachusetts General Hospital (MGH) Department of Psychiatry, was the study's lead author.

Earlier in 2009, the American Medical Association's, American Medical News* (vol. 59, #9) includes an article: *"The long goodbye: The challenge of discontinuing antidepressants; Tapering slowly is the mantra for pruning these regimens, but some patients may still experience withdrawal symptoms."*

- *"For various reasons, patients often are eager to discontinue antidepressants."*

    - *"Some stop or reduce dosages on their own because of side effects, the expense, a desire not to take pills anymore or as a response to perceived stigma."*

    - The labels of antidepressants warn of symptoms that can occur with sudden discontinuation, and physicians often use this as a motivator for adherence.

    - Studies suggest about 20% of patients on these

medications will experience symptoms of what's been coined "the antidepressant discontinuation syndrome" when they try to stop.

- Only a fraction of antidepressant side effects are reported to the FDA. The 20% experiencing withdrawal may actually be quite higher.

- Some patients may be traumatized by the discontinuation attempt.

Dr. Charles Whitfield M.D., describes in detail the trauma caused by psychoactive medications in his new book, Not Crazy: You May Not Be Mentally Ill. Many times we spend more time assisting a person through the trauma caused by these medications than the actual withdrawal of the drug. This is also the part where the real you begins to come out and shine again. The Road Back Program does handle the body and the drug now with ease and this can be quite shocking for some individuals. If you were to take a person who has never spoken one word and have them speak overnight, if you were to take any person addicted to a drug and create such a sweeping positive change in a matter of hours, they need time to adjust and get accustom to how they now feel. This feeling has been described to me as near overwhelming and has been instrumental in helping overcome the drug-induced trauma.

I have included information from these two articles in this section of the book for a few reasons:

1. I want you to know you are not alone with how you may feel now and that your experience with attempting to get off an antidepressant in the past was not you being mentally ill.

2. There are risks with antidepressants that may be downplayed

by your physician. Your physician may not even be aware of the two studies I have mentioned. Educate yourself.

Review the chapter, Medication Side Effects Defined for a complete list of published side effects of psychoactive medication.

My intent is not to worry you, but to inform. Each physician, before prescribing any medication is required to use what is called Informed Consent. Explaining the risk and benefits in a manner that the patient can fully understand, is Informed Consent. This list of side effects includes the risks associated with stopping any medication. In other words, the side effects that are possible while taking the medication can also happen during withdrawal from the drug. All too often, a person was able to use an antidepressant for years and never gain weight, but the moment they began to reduce the antidepressant weight gain started. This weight gain was a withdrawal side effect.

The Final Stages of The Road Back Program

While I start to write this part of the book I am overwhelmed with emotion. This has been a fourteen-year journey so far and most of my original goals with this program have now reached their conclusion. I almost wish I could now sit back and relax and put my attention elsewhere, but it is time to set the next goals for this program and ensure they are as far reaching as they were in 1999.

It is equally as important for you to begin setting your next goals as you read this book. You will get off the medication and you will feel good once again and there will be a reach for life. Getting off the medication is a major decision and will feel like a major accomplishment and having your next goal ready to launch is vital. Don't let any person tell you that you can't attain your new goal. What have you dreamt of doing for years? Start planning now!

In June 2010, I happened on a clinical study detailing the cause of antidepressant weight gain. We have a gene in our body that is called JNK, and the JNK gene becomes over activated by antidepressants and that phenomenon is the cause of antidepressant induced weight gain. On further research I found the activation of the JNK gene is not only the cause of antidepressant induced weight gain, but virtually all side effects caused by a psychoactive medication can be directly linked to the over activation of the JNK gene. Reducing the JNK gene expression can be accomplished naturally and that technique is now a major part of this program.

The role of the JNK gene in our health is a basic starting point. Most disease cannot begin or at the least cause harm inside the body unless this JNK gene becomes overly activated. The Poliovirus must first activate the JNK gene, Parkinson's does not begin until the JNK gene is stimulated, and cancer and tumors cannot exist as long as the JNK gene remains in a normal state. An autistic begins to lose their symptoms of autism when this JNK gene expression is reduced. Diabetes requires an activated JNK gene, just the same as weight gain and liver conditions.

Asian's have a problem when consuming alcohol due to a missing gene. When an Asian drinks alcohol, the alcohol creates an immediate and prolonged activation of the JNK gene and this is what causes the near immediate intoxication, liver problems and more.

The answer is to reduce the JNK gene activation naturally and quickly. This is what The Road Back Program now accomplishes. This may seem like this program is treating, preventing or curing disease with these statements, we are not.

We are just reducing the activation of the JNK gene and

letting the body do what it naturally does when this gene is regulated effectively.

Drugs create a metabolic disorder. The metabolic disorder occurs while taking the drug as well as when you begin reducing the drug. An example of one would be the depletion of the B vitamin biotin if a person has a prolonged use of a benzodiazepine, anti-anxiety drug. The individual may experience a reaction to bright light, a reaction to loud noise and more. This is a symptom of low biotin in the body and when you take biotin the symptom goes away as long as it was coming from low biotin levels. This approach is not treating, preventing or curing an illness or disease.

In closing, as you read this book, perhaps you might be thinking "...this sounds good for others..." or "...others can make it, but not me..." Believe me; I am referring directly to you.

My best to you in your journey,

Jim Harper

Dedication

To my mother, I thank you from the bottom of my heart. As a child you gave me a safe space to just be a child and allowed me to stumble and learn from my mistakes. As an adult you encouraged me to keep looking for new answers. With your passing this past year you have helped me learn value in each moment. Thank you and you are missed.

To my love, best friend and wife. This book would never have been written without you. This program would never have been developed without you. Your insistence in the early days is why The Road Back Program is here. Thank you.

To all of you that have helped along the way, your assistance has been invaluable.

Dr. Hyla Cass M.D., your years of lecturing and helping others are beyond compare and thank you for reviewing this book.

Chapter 1

The Road Back Basics

THE ROAD BACK Program is a very specific, heavily researched, proven program. This program is designed to help people get off all types of psychoactive medications, while reducing to almost zero the crippling side effects often associated with coming off the medication. With the recent advancements of this program, many people are now using the principles of this program for their general health, even if they have never used drugs or medications. The basics of the body are the same whether medication withdrawal is your goal or not and the same successes are available.

Newly formulated psychoactive medications seem to incessantly roll out of research labs into distribution. Nevertheless, we have found over the years that no matter what the drug's formulation, The Road Back Program is still effective. Since you are reading this book you most likely understand, firsthand, the side effects that are possible with psychoactive medications and are looking for real answers.

Which Side Effects Are You Suffering From?

Due to the widely varying circumstances of the many people who will read this book, we have outlined several scenarios delineating where you might now stand, and how The Road Back Program will apply to you.

If you are not on a medication, read through the chapters of this book. This will increase your understanding of what is probably happening within your body and guide you through steps you can take for general health, as well as, what you can do to eliminate anxiety, depression, insomnia and a host of conditions.

Many of you are in the middle of withdrawal when you find this book. We want you to know, how you feel can be remedied and this can be accomplished quickly. Read all chapters of the book and feel free to contact us at The Road Back for guidance. Pay close attention to the chapter, What to Do if You Are Already in Withdrawal or Quit Your Medication Cold Turkey if that applies to you.

If you are on a medication and have not started to taper yet, take your time, read through the material found in this book, get with your prescribing physician and have your full taper plan in place.

If you are already off a drug or medication and an extended period of time has passed, The Road Back Program can still assist. This scenario is often referred to as "protracted withdrawal." You may be sensitive to most supplements and foods by now and completely on edge. The Road Back Program should still be of benefit, it may take a little tweaking and we do suggest you contact us for an individualized program.

I urge you to not give up hope. This program should get you fully recovered from the medication.

You can send us an e-mail as well to info@theroadback.org and we will help guide you through the program.

Chapter 2

The Four Simple Steps

STEP ONE

Do Not Stop Your Medications Abruptly

- Do not "self-medicate" (adjust the medication dosage without consulting your prescribing physician).

- Do not think you are somehow "different" regarding your medications and think you can cut your medications by 50%, or skip days of the medication, etc.

- Keep it simple; follow the program.

- If you are doing well and seeing results, do not change anything. Just stay on the program.

- Remember that The Road Back Program is a systematic process.

STEP TWO

Find Out What You Will Need for the Program

- Read through the Pre-Taper chapter for your medication or situation.

STEP THREE

Get a Complete Physical

- Schedule a complete physical with your doctor.

  Take this book with you and review the program with your doctor.

- Have your physician rule out any actual physical illness or disease.

STEP FOUR

- Purchase Your Supplements and Get Started
- Go to www.Shop.NeuroGeneticSolutions.com and locate a distributor nearest you and purchase the supplements needed for your personal program.

Chapter 3

"Nutritionals" Used
On The Road Back
Program

Disclosure: : I want you to know before you read this chapter, I own the company, Neuro Genetic Solutions, which manufactures most of the supplements used in The Road Back Program. It is important for the supplements to be continually manufactured exactly as I have formulated them, and I have found that the **only** way to insure that all of the products used in The Road Back Program are of the highest quality and effectiveness, is to oversee this process myself. My goal is to maintain these standards for higher quality ingredients while also working to ensure that they are as affordable as possible.

In 1999, we were assisting individuals off their medication without using nutritional supplements by having people gradually reduce the dosage. We came up with a slow tapering process, wherein the drug was only tapered further when a person felt they could handle the withdrawal side effects caused by the previous taper of the medication. Roughly 50% of the people could taper off their medication using a gradual taper, but the 50% that successfully got off their medication still suffered extreme withdrawal side effects. The F.D.A. and the drug companies now recommend what we were doing in 1999, with a gradual reduction.

However, we were not satisfied with a 50% success rate or with the suffering that still took place during the taper process for the lucky half that could get off their medication. We began experimenting with a few nutritional supplements in 2001 to see if they would help with the side effects, and the success rate increased enough for further investigation.

In 2004 I started a DNA testing company and we conducted hundreds of DNA test on individuals who were either currently taking medication, off their medication already or had never used a psychoactive medication.

We looked at how our individual DNA altered the metabolism of drugs as well as how we were able to metabolize food groups and specific nutrients. This information made it very clear why some people experienced adverse reactions to their drug immediately and why some were able to take the drug for an extended period of time before having a negative reaction. However, the DNA Drug Reaction Test did not give evidence or become useful with how to get a person off a drug. The DNA testing of food groups and nutrients did show promise. With this information, we began to create nutritional formulations in the hope it would help eliminate withdrawal side effects or at the least reduce them to a livable amount.

Although the steps above were complicated to a degree, the real work was to create formulations of supplements that would not interact with drugs and would reduce or eliminate side effects associated with tapering off psychoactive medication. At the time, this was unchartered territory in the scientific community, but with our research and success we now see our discoveries and breakthroughs used by many physicians and drug detoxification programs throughout the world.

The nutritional supplements used with The Road Back Program have changed over the past decade as new discoveries have become known. The spring of 2013, has brought the next generation of research to application. Over the past decade, I have spent thousands of hours researching the correct and most basic nutrient system for this program. This edition of the book makes the program even more effective, easier to follow and dramatically reduces the time it takes to get off psychoactive medications. Our goal is and always will be to get a person feeling better faster and allow an individual to safely reduce their medication in less time.

The breakthrough this spring 2013, deals with the time release medications, benzodiazepines and antipsychotic medications. Most new antidepressants are only available as a time release and antipsychotic medications are quickly following suit. The time release drug could not be reduced slow enough to reduce the risk of withdrawal side effects. Often, the individual would need to go back up on the dosage and would never attempt to taper the drug again, even with encouragement from the prescribing physician to reduce the medication.

When the body's chemistry or systems are altered, the body will fight back to balance out the attack. Bringing back that balance is critical if a person is taking a psychoactive medication or if they are suffering from the feeling of anxiety, stress or depression without ever having taken a psychoactive drug.

This program is based on clinical studies conducted by major universities and scientific bodies kept in high regard by the medical community. Here are a few of the results of clinical studies used while developing this program: Antidepressants cause insulin resistance, and if you are predisposed to diabetes and take an antidepressant, you have a four-fold increased chance of becoming a diabetic. Prolonged use of benzodiazepines depletes the body of the B vitamin biotin and can cause problems with receptors used by a benzodiazepine. These two examples give an indication of how one might treat medication side effects and why a few supplements are part of this program.

In other words, if you have taken a benzodiazepine for an extended period of time and have depression and/or tingling or numbness of the extremities, you are probably deficient in biotin. Thus, adding biotin to your daily routine will usually handle the symptom if the biotin deficiency is, in fact, the cause.

The list of symptoms associated with insulin resistance is quite long. Diabetes and obesity are two of several conditions resulting from insulin resistance, but there are other symptoms a person will begin experiencing before the onset of such conditions. Antidepressants cause these body conditions and consequently create physical symptoms that can be confused with actual drug withdrawal symptoms, making the withdrawal from any drug more confusing for the individual and their physician.

How the Program Works

Your body naturally triggers a self-protective inflammatory process when a psychoactive medication is started. This natural function also responds to normal activities, such as exercise, fighting off toxins, allergies, illness, incorrect foods, weight gain, medications, you name it.

For example, let's take a sore throat or an infected cut. The area becomes red and inflamed as the body rushes microscopic "fire fighters" to the area to contain and put out the fire and start the healing process.

However, if your body gets overloaded and can no longer control the inflammation or lacks enough "fire fighters" to douse the flames, then an internal switch flips, and your systems will start going awry, ultimately resulting in an overall imbalance. At this point, but probably earlier in the process, a gene called JNK that is found in all of our cells becomes over activated. If you are taking a drug, there is no doubt the JNK gene is now over activated. This over activation of the JNK gene is the underlying cause of side effects and bodily and mental symptoms associated with all psychoactive drugs.

If you have a physical condition, including menopause, weight gain, diabetes or so many others, and then throw psychoactive medications on top, you can be adding fuel to an already burning fire. In essence, you flip the switch that overloads your body so it can no longer function as intended.

However, and a big however, using supplements (specifically antioxidants) incorrectly, in the wrong amount, combination or time of day, can cause more harm than help.

Reducing the over activation of the JNK gene and cleaning up the cause/effect phenomena is what gives you relief from the drug side effects, allowing the body to heal itself.

The body will produce and release substances called cytokines when the immune system is activated. When the JNK gene becomes over activated, the immune system will begin to have difficulty handling the body and a protein called Interleukin-2 will either plummet or shoot sky high. High Interleukin-2 levels will create a mania in an individual. A chronic high Interleukin-2 will also cause a different substance called Interleukin-6 to become high, and a high level of Interleukin-6 is associated with depression. It is now known, high Interleukin-6 precedes depressions. Here you have the bipolar individual who cycles between mania and depression.

Depending on your body and what you were exposed to, these cytokines may have been overly active before you started taking medication, or they may have become inhibited once the medication was started. We all react differently when medication is taken. One thing is common with all of us—the need to maintain or get back to a natural body balance.

Oxidative stress will be significantly higher in the body of anyone diagnosed with anxiety, depression, bipolar, schizophrenia, ADHD and OCD. The brain is most susceptible to oxidative stress, and a multitude of clinical trials have shown *significantly higher oxidative stress in the brain of bipolar and schizophrenic patients.* The supplements called Neuro Endure and JNK will help stop the oxidative stress before it even starts or stop the continued progress if it is already underway.

The area of nutrition is littered with confusing words and information so technical it can seem overwhelming. I have tried to simplify and distill what you need to know so you can proceed with the program while understanding the basic premise of how your body works to counteract the imbalances created by the medication.

If you wish to read more of the technical information please read the Science chapter.

Thousands of people worldwide have stood where you now stand-ready to take their lives back and free themselves from psychoactive medication and the resulting side effects. While every person is unique and life offers no guarantees, if you follow this program precisely, you should begin to feel better soon after you start.

Supplements Used in the Program

The supplements used with The Road Back Program are manufactured by **Neuro Genetic Solutions** (Neuro Endure Mini, JNK Capsules, Omega 3 Supreme – TG, Body Calm Daytime Relief, Body Calm Supreme With Melatonin, Body Calm Supreme Melatonin Free and Adrenalpin), **Transfer Point** (Beta 1-3 D Glucan) and **A.C. Grace** (Unique E). The chapters in this book that detail how to taper specific types of medication will list which supplements you need to use for each drug type as well as additional supplements to use for more specific withdrawal symptoms. This chapter describes all supplements that might be used in the program and gives tips on how to use each one.

Adrenalpin – (Manufactured by Neuro Genetic Solutions) Adrenalpin should be used, no matter the drug you may be taking if; when you awake in the morning you feel anxiety, the feeling tends to reduce a little as noontime approaches but then comes back again full force near noon. The anxiety feeling will usually fade again a little as the day passes and in the evening, if you are not able to be asleep by 10:30pm the anxiety feeling comes back fully and you are not able to go to sleep until after 1am.

Adrenalpin is formulated with Cordyceps (mushroom), Eleuthero, Rhodiola, Montmorency Tart Cherry and Pantothenic Acid. This formula is made to slowly reduce the feeling of daytime anxiety and help with sleep. There are more direct ways to adjust the body to eliminate the anxiety feelings but the approach is too harsh and even if you have never used a psychoactive medication those other supplements would cause you to have an increased anxiety and insomnia.

This is where even a good Naturopathic Doctor may error in the treatment of a patient on psychoactive medication. They have a formula they have used for years and it has been very effective and they feel it will be fine with most of their patients. If you are taking anti-anxiety drug this definitely is not the case. If you were prescribed an antidepressant for anxiety, it probably will cause more harm than help as well.

Slow and steady wins the race, especially with the feeling of anxiety.

You should take 2 capsules of the Adrenalpin each day with food. Take the first capsule in the morning and the second capsule about 30-minutes before the normal return of the anxiety feeling near noon. Make sure to have some food in the stomach each time you take Adrenalpin.

The Adrenalpin veggie capsules are guaranteed to dissolve within 15-minutes after swallowing.

B6, B12 and Folate – You should be able to find a B6, B12 and Folate at a local vitamin store. The supplement should be made from: Vitamin B6 (from pyridoxal 5'-phosphate) Folate (50% as folinic acid (5-formyltetrahydrofolate) and 50% as 5-methyltetrahydroflate) and B12 (as methylcobalamin).

Approximately, 30% of the population will not be able to metabolize B12 and folate with ease. If you do not use the types mentioned here, the chances of metabolism reduce further.

If you have difficulty finding a supplement exactly as described, Dr. Hyla Cass M.D. offers a multi-vitamin on her web site that will be close enough. Her site address is www.cassmd.com and the multi is called Two a Day Better Balance Multi.

Before you just use any multi-vitamin, check the label and see if the folate reads folic acid. If so, this is a synthetic folate and will actually mutate your genes instead of providing help to the body.

Taking a B6, B12 and Folate should not cause any reaction at all. Low folate levels are common with depression and we do not get enough folate in our diet, especially when 30% of us have a difficult time metabolizing it in the first place.

Beta 1, 3-D Glucan – This supplement is available from Transfer Point (www.transferpoint.com). The human immune system includes a substance called IL-2. Individuals with low levels of IL-2

13

have anxiety and problems with sleep. Stage 2 of sleep requires a sufficient level of IL-2 for a deep restful sleep.

Beta 1, 3-D Glucan has been clinically proven to not only increase levels of IL-2 in the human immune system but to also keep the IL-2 levels increased for an extended time after the product is discontinued.

If you have anxiety and or insomnia, use the JNK supplement, Body Calm Daytime Relief, Body Calm Supreme and Adrenalpin first. If these symptoms do not completely subside within 2 weeks, you may have low IL-2, and supplementing with the Beta 1, 3-D Glucan would be in order. Taking one or two of the 100 mg capsules in the morning will usually do the trick.

Tip: The Beta 1, 3-D Glucan must be taken apart from food or water and not within a half hour of consuming food or liquid. Only use enough liquid to get the Beta 1, 3-D Glucan down the throat and no more than that. The Beta 1, 3-D Glucan needs to absorb, and taking it in any other fashion will not allow assimilation.

JNK Capsules – (Manufactured by Neuro Genetic Solutions) The JNK has been reformulated to be close to the original formula from 2010. This was the most effective formula in this program, hands down. As new clinical studies were published about the individual ingredients in the formula it became apparent why it was more effective. The JNK Capsules are back!

The ingredients in the JNK Capsule are; Milk Thistle, Selenium, N-Acetyl-Cysteine, Alpha Lipoic Acid, Biotin, Inositol, Malic Acid, Calcium as citrate malate, Alpha Ketoglutaric Acid, Vitamin K2 as menaquinone-7, and

Pantothenic Acid.

Milk Thistle helps reduce the over activation of the JNK gene. The amount used in this supplement will not give much help to the liver. That is not the purpose of the Milk Thistle in this formula.

The Selenium helps reduce the over activation of the JNK gene plus it helps support normal cell health and has a specific antioxidant action.

N-Acetyl-Cysteine (NAC) creates the master antioxidant glutathione. NAC is the most heavily researched product regarding glutathione. For this reason, you will find NAC used in emergency rooms as an IV treatment and prescribed by physicians for various reasons.

NAC does help reduce the over activation of the JNK gene and works hand-in-hand with selenium, alpha lipoic acid, vitamin C and vitamin E. NAC will have an effect within the brain and liver.

Alpha Lipoic Acid helps recirculate vitamin C and vitamin E and has a distinct benefit with insulin resistance. It is normally never used as a standalone supplement but is a supporting cast member that wins best supporting actor at the Oscars each and every year.

Biotin is usually thought of for hair and nail problems. Anti-anxiety drugs deplete biotin with prolonged usage of the drug and you may have brittle hair and nails. Those are only the possible visible signs. Numbness or tingling of the extremities occurs when the drugs have depleted biotin too much. I increased the biotin in this formula to be higher than what was found in the original JNK.

Inositol is a key cell membrane component and messenger in our neuro-communication system. It signals the release of serotonin and norepinephrine. It also triggers other cellular functions, such as glucose and fat metabolism. With insulin resistance being a major underlying problem with most people taking a psychoactive drug, the more help for that area the better.

The amount of inositol in the JNK Capsule formula is not enough to stop taking inositol if you are already doing so. The amount used is just enough to be effective with the overall formula.

Malic Acid is a supplement most people have never heard of. Malic acid is used for making ATP, which is a molecule that provides energy to muscles, brain, heart and other tissues.

Calcium, as calcium citrate malate. It is all too common for people doing this program to have the feelings associated with anxiety. Part of the physical reason can come from calcium. Calcium can excite the body rather much, to put it mildly. I have found calcium citrate does not cause this agitation but also works to calm things down. Many of us also have the genetic makeup that makes absorption of calcium difficult. I have used calcium citrate malate in the formula to give a high bioavailability of a well absorbed calcium. If you are taking a calcium supplement already, I want you to know there is 254mg of calcium citrate malate in each serving of the JNK formula. There are 3 capsules to a serving.

Alpha Ketoglutaric Acid (AKG) is another one of those supplements you probably never heard anything about. This supplement helps remove ammonia from the central nervous system.

This is an organic acid that helps metabolism of all essential amino acids and assist with the transfer of cellular energy in the citric acid cycle. The body needs AKG as a precursor to glutamic acid, which is involved in protein synthesis and the regulation of blood glucose levels.

A buildup of ammonia in the brain, muscles and kidneys can occur with psychoactive drug usage. This is part of the reason the list of drug side effects included these areas of the body.

Vitamin K2 as menaquinone-7 is from a natural source. Vitamin K2 has a role in blood coagulation, a benefit for bone health and vascular function. This form of K2 also has the longest half-life of all K2 vitamins making it suitable for this formula.

This form of K2 has been shown to help reduce bone loss in postmenopausal women.

For those of you taking a blood thinner, the amount of K2 in each capsule is 16mcg. Please share this with your physician before taking the JNK Capsules.

Pantothenic Acid is an essential B vitamin that is needed to release energy from carbohydrates, protein and fats from food. It is also essential for the synthesis of adrenal hormones and cholesterol. This supplement is also involved in fatty acid metabolism and many of the enzyme processes of the body.

The biotin mentioned earlier, also requires pantothenic acid to be the most effective.

You will also find pantothenic acid in the Adrenalpin formula. I have kept in mind you may be taking both the Adrenalpin and the JNK Capsules and have formulated both products in such a manner so you will not have too much pantothenic acid.

The JNK Capsules are guaranteed to dissolve within 15-minutes after swallowing.

Neuro Endure and Neuro Endure Mini – Start off with the Neuro Endure Mini. The Mini is the same formula as Neuro Endure but with ¼ the strength. Most of you will only need the Neuro Endure Mini. This product was formulated to help those of you taking a timed release medication but it was found to be very effective with benzodiazepines and other drugs as well.

In testing the key ingredients of this supplement, a few things happened that were surprising. People with protracted withdrawal had symptoms leave in a manner of days. There were people that usually could not take any supplement due to adverse reactions.

Don't be surprised if your, anxiety, insomnia, memory and concentration returns or improves. It is common for relief from body aches and pains to diminish with Neuro Endure.

Unless you are tapering from a pain medication, start with the Neuro Endure Mini. I detail how to take in the Pre-taper chapters.

The ingredients in Neuro Endure are; Acetyl-L-Carnitine, Bacopa Monnieri, L-Glutamine and N-Acetyl-Cysteine.

Acetyl-L-Carnitine reduces the over activation of the JNK gene in the brain. This is probably why this supplement has been used by physicians to help with brain and nerve function during aging. This ingredient is a metabolic source for acetylcholine, a brain neurotransmitter and with the conversion back to L-Carnitine; it helps carry fatty acids into the mitochondria of nerve, heart and muscle cells for the production of energy. Other benefits include; cell membrane stability, production of nerve growth factor

18

and cerebral blood flow.

Bacopa Monnieri is an herb that has been used for centuries to help with mood. The amount of the herb in this formula matches the amount and strength used in the successful studies.

L-Glutamine is a primary source of energy for intestinal immune cells and a major amino acid in muscle tissue. With continual stress, the body loses the ability to manufacture enough glutamine naturally and supplementation is required.

N-Acetyl-Cysteine. Please see description of this supplement in the description of the JNK Capsules.

The Neuro Endue Mini tablets are guaranteed to dissolve within 30-minutes after swallowing.

Omega 3 Supreme TG – (Manufactured by Neuro Genetic Solutions) This omega 3 is completely a new omega 3 fish oil for The Road Back Program. With redoing the manufacturing of products used in the program, I knew the omega 3 fish oil could be upgraded to a better product. Starting from scratch, and looking at what role a fish oil has in this program; that being to assist with the "brain zaps" associated with reducing an antidepressant, a new type of fish oil was selected.

Other than the cheap, run-of-the-mill fish oil, a distillation process is used to purify the fish oil and remove heavy metals and toxins that are present in fish. All omega 3's we recommended in the past were distilled.

During the distillation process, alcohols are used to help breakdown the fish oil and purify it. This is the time when you can increase the amount of EPA in the fish oil or the DHA fraction. If you look at the back of any fish oil label you will see EPA in milligrams, DHA stated in milligrams, as well as total milligrams of fatty acids. This

19

is the point where nearly all fish oil processing stops due to price and you have a fish oil product called EE or ethyl esters. If the bottle of fish oil you have on your shelf does not state TG on the label, it is undoubtedly this EE form.

The EE form is not a natural form for fish oil. It is still in an altered state and not natural. Synthetic if you will.

The Omega 3 Supreme is in the TG form of fish oil. The manufacturing process for TG fish oil takes the fish oil back to the natural structure of fish oil. The human body likes natural! It knows what to do with things that are natural.

The TG stands for triglyceride. A natural omega 3 is in the triglyceride form, not the EE form.

The triglyceride in omega 3 fish oil is not the same as triglyceride as a "fat" you may want to be lowering under your doctor's care. A completely different animal!

If you have experienced burping, the fish breathe, you have been taking the EE form of fish oil.

If you do much research on the difference between EE and TG fish oil, you will find most clinical studies have used the EE form of fish oil. That is because it is cheaper.

Once the fish oil is ready to convert back to the TG form, a choice is made on how much EPA/DHA the product will have. You will find some fish oil in TG form to have around 180mg of EPA and a low amount of DHA as well. This is great for a child as long as the total amount of fish oil is still not at 1,000mg a softgel.

Omega 3 Supreme TG has 408mg of EPA, 272mg of DHA, 70mg of other fatty acids per softgel. In the future, as new batches of the Omega 3 Supreme TG are made, the amount of EPA, DHA and total other fatty acids may go up or down slightly. The manufacturing process for fish oils is not the same as making a vitamin C where the milligram amount can be exact each time. The product is made with the same procedures, the product is then tested and measured and the exact amount must be on each label.

The cost is higher per softgel of TG omega 3 as compared to the EE form. However, the high host averages out when you compare the amount of TG softgels you will need to take is less. With TG being in a natural state, the omega 3 fish oil has over 30% higher absorption.

The next 3 supplements are where quality and price have been addressed.

Body Calm Daytime Relief – (Manufactured by Neuro Genetic Solutions)

Body Calm Daytime Relief is formulated to be used during the daytime to help with relief from anxiety. If you are responding quite well to this supplement during the daytime you may want to try it at bedtime as well for sleep.

The Montmorency tart cherry is without binders or fillers from the supplier, passion flower is pure and at a good strength, L-Theanine and 50mg of GABA.

I was the first to recommend the Montmorency cherry for anxiety and sleep back in 2004. You may find other cherry supplements now recommended for these symptoms and if they did not work for you don't think this supplement will not. Using a pure cherry powder, including the skin, without binders makes a huge difference in this product.

21

Using these supplements are different than most other supplements you might have used for anxiety or sleep. They do not make you drowsy or sleepy.

The Body Calm Daytime Relief works well when taken together with the Adrenalpin. Getting relief from the daytime feelings of anxiety is essential for a productive day and believe me; a day filled with the feeling of anxiety does get in the way of your sleep. I am probably preaching to the choir here but if you also have a difficult time with sleep, what you do or do not do in the daytime will directly affect how well and how easy you can go to sleep.

The veggie capsules used with Body Calm Daytime Relief are guaranteed to dissolve within 15-minutes after swallowing.

Body Calm Supreme Melatonin Free – (Manufactured by Neuro Genetic Solutions) When you take this supplement 15-minutes before bedtime the capsule will dissolve right as you go to bed. Don't expect to feel sleepy suddenly. Close your eyes and start going to sleep and don't be surprised if you just awake the next morning.

Body Calm Supreme Melatonin Free includes a blend of Montmorency tart cherry, passion flower, L-Theanine and GABA. If you compare the formula of Body Calm Daytime Relief and Body Calm Supreme Melatonin Free you will notice the exact same formula. However, the amount of each ingredient has been changed to help guide you through the switchover from the Body Calm Daytime Relief to sleep, without jarring your system. The amount of GABA used in this formula is very low.

One to two capsules 15-minutes before bedtime.

The veggie capsules used with Body Calm Supreme Melatonin Free are guaranteed to dissolve within 15-minutes after swallowing.

Body Calm Supreme With Melatonin – (Manufactured by Neuro Genetic Solutions) This formula is the exact same as the Body Calm Supreme Melatonin Free except for the addition of vitamin B1 as Benfotiamine and melatonin.

Vitamin B1 as Benfotiamine was used because I wanted a B1 that would cross the blood-brain-barrier. Melatonin can cause some people to have vivid nightmares or vivid dreams and B1 has been shown to help.

Take 1 to 2 capsules 15-minutes before bedtime.

The capsule is guaranteed to dissolve within 15-minutes after swallowing.

Unique E – Omega 3 fish oil requires vitamin E for absorption. If you take any omega 3 fish oil daily you will become deficient in vitamin E in time. I have recommended the Unique E made by A.C. Grace Company for years. A.C. Grace has been making vitamin E for over 50-years and their blend of mixed vitamin E is unique, as their name suggest. It is a natural blend of the parts that make up vitamin E. Neuro Genetic Solutions will probably carry the Unique E so you do not need to shop at multiple web sites. If you would prefer to purchase directly from A.C. Grace, their web site is www.acgrace.com.

A recap on where the supplements are available.

Neuro Genetic Solutions – Adrenalpin, JNK Capsules, Neuro Endure, Neuro Endure Mini, Omega 3 Supreme TG, Body Calm

Daytime Relief, Body Calm Supreme Melatonin Free, Body Calm Supreme With Melatonin

www.shop.neurogeneticsolutions.com

Neuro Genetic Solutions is based in the United States and has distributors in Europe, Australia, and Canada and very soon in Hong Kong. Go to www.shop.neurogeneticsolutions.com for distributor web site information.

Beta 1-3D Glucan – Is available at www.transferpoint.com

Chapter 4

Drug Side Effects

Side Effects of Psychoactive Medications

This book addresses drugs of all types. The drugs we are dealing with are usually classified as psychotropic – having ability or quality of altering emotions, perceptions, behaviors, and bodily functions – especially true of certain drugs.

This chapter lists many possible side effects experienced from either taking these drugs, or when trying to withdraw from them. If you, or anyone you know, are taking any of these drugs the "real you" could well be buried under some of the following symptoms. But rest assured, no one has all of these side effects, and no single drug or combination of these drugs can produce all the side effects listed here.

You may know from experience that a single withdrawal side effect can be horrifying. And if you, or anyone you know, have ever had a bad withdrawal experience you would probably rather sign up for open-heart surgery without anesthesia than suffer those side effects again. And for this very reason, many people who have contacted The Road Back Program are gun shy at the very thought of withdrawing from a drug. Before The Road Back Program, you were faced with a quandary: suffer the side effects of the drugs, or gut it out and suffer the side effects of withdrawal.

One thing to keep in mind while doing this program or with any inpatient program you might enroll in, if you have a bad day and feel out of sorts, have a headache, an ache or a pain, do not sleep well etc., these feelings or symptoms may not be withdrawal. We all have bad days from time to time and how you feel out of the blue can be quite normal. This can be difficult when you have had insomnia for months and begin to sleep better and then out of the blue you have a difficult night sleeping. If the insomnia last for more than 3 nights then something needs to be done, but an occasional restless night or sleepless night is common.

This past year we had a person call us and she described how she has had a headache for the past 4 days and how it came out of nowhere. She was ½ way off her medication and doing very well and she felt this was a withdrawal side effect and wanted to know what to do. After a little communication and looking for changes that might have taken place, we found out her best friend had died unexpectedly the day before the headaches started. This might seem easy to spot as a reason for the headaches, but when you are in the middle of withdrawal and you have suffered extreme withdrawal side effects in the past, it can be easy to lose track and worry about the slightest changes in how you feel.

As you read through the list of side effects in this chapter, do keep in mind these emotional and physical conditions existed long before the first psychoactive drug was manufactured. We are only dealing with drug induced side effects with this program.

The Road Back Program helps to eliminate these worries and concerns by reducing the side effects of withdrawal, so that you can come off your drug(s) smoothly and easily.

The following list is broken down into categories, covering the various areas of the body, such as the nervous system, lymph system, emotional and mental symptoms and so forth. These categories will make it easier for you to find the part of the body or system that you are interested in, or want to know more about.

In this list, you will find many physical ailments and complaints, as well as emotional or mental symptoms that people experience every day because of a specific medical condition. These symptoms and ailments may be the reason that you started using a drug, or conversely, these drugs may actually be causing the negative symptoms you are experiencing now.

This unknown catches almost everyone, doctor and patient alike, off guard. So the question that needs to be answered, in order for you to proceed with The Road Back Program is: Are you dealing with a physical condition that needs to be treated medically or with a by-product symptom of the drug(s) you are taking?

Getting Your Doctor's Approval

Because of the overload and damage potentially caused by drugs, your body in general, and your immune system in particular, are in a weakened condition, and can thus leave you open to infections and disease. On the other hand, you may be taking prescription medications for actual physical conditions, which could be contra-indicated or need to be closely monitored in terms of doing The Road Back Program. These could include blood thinners and heart medication, as well as clotting agents.

For these reasons, consult your doctor before starting any part of this program to sort out, or discover and correctly determine, whether you are a candidate for The Road Back Program.

27

After you have ruled out any real medical problem, you will know that if any strange symptom begins during The Road Back Program, you are most likely experiencing something caused by the drug you are taking. Such will be true for both emotional and physical symptoms.

Antidepressants, antipsychotics, anti-anxiety drugs give such a broad side effect profile, the list of side effects in this chapter are side effects with those drugs. You may be taking a pain killer, hypnotic, alcohol or street drugs, but if you go through the list of side effects in this chapter you will find you have more than a few. The reason the side effects from psychoactive medications mimic other drug side effects is due to what was discussed in earlier chapters and the science chapter, that being, the activation of the JNK gene and the need for an adaptogen to come in and clean up the havoc created by the drug.

The following list does not include all possible side effects from drugs, this book would need thousands of pages if this were undertaken. Using the Freedom of Information Act, I received all side effects associated with a popular antidepressant medication during clinical trials. That list alone is long enough to make this book be double the size if they were included. The side effects in this chapter are the most common.

The list of side effects in the first part of this chapter are for antidepressants, antipsychotics and ADHD medications. Later in this chapter you will find benzodiazepine, anti-anxiety and sleep medication/ narcotics/hypnotics side

28

effects.

SIDE EFFECTS OF ANTIDEPRESSANTS, ANTIPSYCHOTICS AND ADHD MEDICATION GENERAL BODY

Dry Mouth - Less moisture in the mouth than is usual.

Increased Sweating - A large quantity of perspiration that is medically caused.

Allergy - Extreme sensitivity of body tissues triggered by substances in the air, drugs, or foods causing a variety of reactions such as sneezing, itching, asthma, hay fever, skin rashes, nausea and/or vomiting.

Asthenia - A physically weak condition.

Chest Pains - Severe discomfort in the chest caused by not enough oxygen going to the heart because of blood vessel narrowing or spasms.

Chills - Appearing pale while cold and shivering. Sometimes accompanied by fever.

Edema of Extremities - Abnormal swelling of body tissue caused by the collection of fluid.

Fall - Suddenly losing a normal standing upright position.

Fatigue - Loss of normal strength thus not able to do usual physical and mental activities.

Fever - Abnormally high body temperature, normal being 98.6 degrees Fahrenheit or 37 degrees Centigrade. Fever is a symptom of disease or disorder in the body. The body is affected by feeling hot, chilled, sweaty, weak and exhausted. If the fever goes too high or lasts too long, death can result.

Hot Flashes - Brief, abnormal enlargement of the blood vessels that causes a sudden heat sensation over the entire body. Sometimes experienced by menopausal women.

Influenza (Flu)-like Symptoms - Demonstrating irritation of the respiratory tract (organs of breathing) such as a cold, sudden fever, aches and pains, as well as feeling weak and seeking bed rest, which is similar to having the flu.

Leg Pain - A hurtful sensation in the legs caused by excessive stimulation of the nerve endings in the legs, resulting in extreme discomfort.

Malaise - The somewhat unclear feeling of discomfort when a person starts to feel sick.

Pain in Limb - Sudden, sharp and uncontrolled leg or arm discomfort.

Syncope - A short period of light-headedness or unconsciousness (black- out) also known as fainting, caused by lack of oxygen to the brain because of an interruption in blood flow to the brain.

Tightness of Chest - Mild or sharp discomfort, tightness or pressure in the chest area (anywhere between the throat and belly). The causes can be mild or seriously life-threatening because they include the heart, lungs and surrounding muscles.

CARDIOVASCULAR
(INVOLVING THE HEART AND THE BLOOD VESSELS)

Palpitation - Unusual and abnormal heartbeat that is sometimes irregular, but rapid, and forceful thumping or fluttering. It can be brought on by shock, excitement, exertion or medical stimulants. A person is normally unaware of his/her heartbeat.

Hypertension - High blood pressure, a symptom of disease in the blood vessels leading away from the heart. Hypertension is known as the "silent killer." The symptoms are usually not obvious; however, it can lead to damage to the heart, brain, kidneys and eyes, and can even lead to stroke and kidney failure.

Bradycardia - The heart rate is slowed from around 72 beats per minute, which is normal, to below 60 beats per minute in an adult.

Tachycardia - The heart rate speeds up to above 100 beats per minute in an adult. Normal adult heart rate average is 72 beats per minute.

ECG Abnormal - A test called an electrocardiogram (ECG) records the activity of the heart by measuring heartbeats as well as the position and size of the heart's four chambers. An ECG also measures whether there is damage to the heart and the effects of drugs or mechanical devices like a heart pacemaker. When the test is abnormal this means one or more of the following are present: heart disease, defects, beating too fast or too slow, disease of the blood vessels leading from the heart or the heart valves, and/or a past or impending heart attack.

Flushing - Skin all over the body turns red.

Varicose Veins - Unusually swollen veins near the surface of the skin that sometimes appear twisted and knotted, but always enlarged. They are called hemorrhoids when appearing around the rectum. The cause is attributed to hereditary weakness in the veins aggravated by obesity, pregnancy, pressure from standing, aging, etc. Severe cases may develop swelling in the legs, ankles and feet, eczema and/or ulcers in the affected areas.

GASTROINTESTINAL (INVOLVING THE STOMACH AND THE INTESTINES)

Abdominal Cramp/Pain - Sudden, severe, uncontrollable and painful shortening and thickening of the muscles in the belly. The belly includes the stomach, as well as the intestines, liver, kidneys, pancreas, spleen, gall bladder and urinary bladder.

Belching - Noisy release of gas from the stomach through the mouth.

Bloating - Swelling of the belly caused by excessive intestinal gas. **Constipation** - Difficulty in having a bowel movement where the

material in the bowels is hard due to a lack of exercise, fluid intake, or roughage in the diet or due to certain drugs.

Diarrhea - Unusually frequent and excessive runny bowel movements that may result in severe dehydration and shock.

Dyspepsia/Indigestion - The discomfort one may experience after eating. Can be heartburn, gas, nausea, a bellyache or bloating.

Flatulence - More gas than normal in the digestive organs.

Gagging - Involuntary choking and/or involuntary vomiting.

Gastritis - A severe irritation of the mucus lining of the stomach, either short in duration or lasting for a long period of time.

Gastroenteritis - A condition in which the membranes of the stomach and intestines are irritated.

Gastrointestinal Hemorrhage - Excessive internal bleeding in the stomach and intestines.

Gastro Esophageal Reflux - A continuous state where stomach juices flow back into the throat causing acid indigestion and heartburn and possibly injury to the throat.

Heartburn - A burning pain in the area of the breastbone caused by

stomach juices flowing back up into the throat.

Hemorrhoids - Small rounded purplish swollen veins that bleed, itch or are painful and appear around the anus.

Increased Stool Frequency - see "Diarrhea."

Indigestion - Inability to properly consume and absorb food in the digestive tract, causing constipation, nausea, stomachache, gas, swollen belly, pain and general discomfort or sickness.

Nausea - Stomach irritation with a queasy sensation similar to motion sickness and a feeling that one is going to vomit.

Polyposis Gastric - Tumors that grow on stems in the lining of the stomach, which usually become cancerous.

Swallowing Difficulty - A feeling that food is stuck in the throat or upper chest area and won't go down, making it difficult to swallow.

Toothache - Pain in a tooth above and below the gum line.

Vomiting - Involuntarily throwing up the contents of the stomach, usually accompanied by a nauseated, sick feeling just prior to doing so.

HEMIC & LYMPHATIC

(INVOLVING THE BLOOD AND THE CLEAR FLUIDS IN THE TISSUES THAT CONTAIN WHITE BLOOD CELLS)

Anemia - A condition in which the blood is no longer carrying enough oxygen, so the person looks pale and easily gets dizzy, weak and tired. More severely, a person can end up with an abnormal heart, as well as breathing and digestive difficulties.

Bruise - Damage to the skin resulting in a purple-green-yellow skin coloration that is caused by breaking of the blood vessels in the area without breaking the surface of the skin.

Nosebleed - Blood loss from the nose.

Hematoma - Broken blood vessels that cause a swelling in an area on the body.

Lymphadenopathy Cervical - The lymph nodes in the neck, part of the body's immune system, become swollen and enlarged by reacting to the presence of a drug. The swelling is the result of the white blood cells multiplying in order to fight the invasion of the drug.

METABOLIC & NUTRITIONAL
(ENERGY AND HEALTH)

Arthralgia – Sudden sharp nerve pain in one or more joints.

Arthropathy – Joint disease or abnormal joints.

Arthritis - Painfully inflamed and swollen joints. The reddened and swollen condition is brought on by a serious injury or shock to the body either from physical or emotional causes.

Back Discomfort - Severe physical distress in the area from the neck to the pelvis along the backbone.

Bilirubin Increased - Bilirubin is a waste product of the breakdown of old blood cells. Bilirubin is sent to the liver to be made water-soluble so it can be eliminated from the body through emptying the bladder. A drug can interfere with or damage this normal liver function, creating liver disease.

Decreased Weight - Uncontrolled and measured loss of heaviness or weight.

Gout - A severe arthritis condition that is caused by the dumping of a waste product called uric acid into the tissues and joints. It can worsen and cause the body to develop a deformity after going through stages of pain, inflammation, severe tenderness and stiffness.

Hepatic Enzymes Increased - An increase in the amount of paired liver proteins that regulate liver processes causing a condition in which the liver functions abnormally.

Hypercholesterolemia - Too much cholesterol in the blood cells.

Hyperglycemia - An unhealthy amount of sugar in the blood.

Increased Weight - A concentration and storage of fat in the body accumulating over a period of time caused by unhealthy eating patterns, a lack of physical activity, or an inability to process food correctly, which can predispose the body to many disorders and diseases.

Jaw Pain - Pain due to irritation and swelling of the nerves associated with the mouth area where it opens and closes just in front of the ear. Some of the symptoms are: pain when chewing, headaches, loss of balance, stuffy ears or ringing in the ears and teeth grinding.

Jaw Stiffness - The result of squeezing and grinding the teeth while asleep that can cause teeth to deteriorate, as well as the muscles and joints of the jaw.

Joint Stiffness - A loss of free motion and easy flexibility.

Muscle Cramp - When muscles contract uncontrollably without warning and do not relax. The muscles of any body organs can cramp.

Muscle Stiffness - The tightening of muscles making it difficult to bend.

Muscle Weakness - Loss of physical strength.

Myalgia - A general widespread pain and tenderness of the muscles.

Thirst - A strong, unnatural craving for moisture/water in the mouth and throat.

NERVOUS SYSTEM (SENSORY CHANNELS)

Carpal Tunnel Syndrome - A pinched nerve in the wrist that causes pain, tingling, and numbing.

Coordination Abnormal - A lack of normal, harmonious interaction of the parts of the body when it is in motion.

Dizziness - Losing one's balance while feeling unsteady and lightheaded. May lead to fainting.

Disequilibrium - Lack of mental and emotional balance.

Faintness - A temporary condition in which one is likely to become unconscious and fall.

Headache - A sharp or dull persistent pain in the head.

Hyperreflexia - A not normal (abnormal) and involuntary increased response in the tissues connecting the bones to the muscles.

Light-Headed Feeling - An uncontrolled and usually brief loss of consciousness usually caused by a lack of oxygen to the brain.

Migraine - Recurring severe head pain sometimes accompanied by nausea, vomiting, dizziness, flashes or spots before the eyes and ringing in the ears.

Muscle Contractions Involuntary - A spontaneous and uncontrollable tightening reaction of the muscles caused by electrical impulses from the nervous system.

Muscular Tone Increased - Uncontrolled and exaggerated muscle tension. Muscles are normally partially tensed which is what gives muscle tone.

37

Paresthesia - Burning, prickly, itchy, or tingling skin with no obvious or understood physical cause.

Restless Legs - A need to move the legs without any apparent reason. Sometimes there is pain, twitching, jerking, cramping, burning or a creepy-crawly sensation associated with the movements. It worsens when a person is inactive, and can interrupt sleep so one feels the need to move to gain some relief.

Shaking - Uncontrolled quivering and trembling as if one is cold and chilled.

Sluggishness - Lack of alertness and energy, as well as being slow to respond or perform in life.

Tics - A contraction of a muscle causing a repeated movement not under the control of the person, usually on the face or limbs.

Tremor - A nervous and involuntary vibrating or quivering of the body.

Twitching - Sharp, jerky and spastic motion, sometimes with a sharp sudden pain.

Vertigo - A sensation of dizziness with disorientation and confusion.

MENTAL AND EMOTIONAL

Aggravated Nervousness - A progressively worsening, irritated, and troubled state of mind.

Agitation - A suddenly violent and forceful emotionally disturbed state of mind.

Amnesia - Long or short term, partial or full memory loss created by emotional or physical shock, severe illness, or a blow to the head where the person was caused pain and became unconscious.

Anxiety Attack - Sudden and intense feelings of fear, terror, and dread, physically creating shortness of breath, sweating, trembling and heart palpitations.

Apathy - Complete lack of concern or interest for things that ordinarily would be regarded as important or would normally cause concern.

Appetite Decreased - Lack of appetite despite the ordinary caloric demands of living, with a resulting unintentional loss of weight.

Appetite Increased - An unusual hunger causing one to overeat.

Auditory Hallucination - Hearing things without the voices or noises being present.

Bruxism - Grinding and clenching of teeth while sleeping.

Carbohydrate Craving - A drive or craving to eat foods rich in sugar and starches (sweets, snacks and junk foods) that intensifies as the diet becomes more and more unbalanced due to the unbalancing of the proper nutritional requirements of the body.

Concentration Impaired - Unable to easily focus attention for long periods of time.

Confusion - Inability to think clearly or understand, preventing logical decision making.

Crying (Abnormal) - Unusual fits of weeping for short or long periods of time for no apparent reason.

39

Depersonalization - A condition in which one has lost a normal sense of personal identity.

Depression - A hopeless feeling of failure, loss and sadness that can deteriorate into thoughts of death. A very common reaction to or side effect of psychiatric drugs.

Disorientation - A loss of sense of direction, place, time or surroundings, as well as mental confusion regarding one's personal identity.

Dreaming (Abnormal) - Dreaming that leaves a very clear, detailed picture and impression when awake that can last for a long period of time and sometimes be unpleasant.

Emotional Lability - Suddenly breaking out in laughter or crying or doing both without being able to control the outburst of emotion. These episodes are unstable as they are caused by experiences or events that normally would not have this effect on an individual.

Excitability - Uncontrollably responding to stimuli (one's environment).

Feeling Unreal - The awareness that one has an undesirable emotion like fear, but can't seem to shake off the irrational feeling. For example, feeling like one is going crazy, but rationally knowing that it is not true. Resembles experiencing a bad dream and not being able to wake up.

Forgetfulness - Unable to remember what one ordinarily would remember.

Insomnia - Sleeplessness caused by physical stress, mental stress or stimulants, such as coffee or medications, awake when one would ordinarily be able to fall and remain asleep.

Irritability - An abnormal reaction of being annoyed or disturbed in response to a stimulus in the environment.

Jitteriness - Nervous fidgeting without apparent cause.

Lethargy - Mental and physical sluggishness and apathy (a feeling of hopelessness that "nothing can be done") which can deteriorate into an unconscious state resembling deep sleep. A numbed state of mind.

Libido Decreased - An abnormal loss of sexual energy or desire.

Panic Reaction - A sudden, overpowering, chaotic and confused mental state of terror resulting in being doubt-ridden, often accompanied with hyperventilation and extreme anxiety.

Restlessness Aggravated - A constantly worsening troubled state of mind characterized by increased nervousness, inability to relax and quick temper.

Somnolence - Feeling sleepy all the time or having a condition of semi- consciousness.

Suicide Attempt - An unsuccessful deliberate attack on one's own life with the intention of ending it.

Suicidal Tendency - Most likely will attempt to kill oneself.

Tremulousness Nervous - Very jumpy, shaky, and uneasy, while feeling fearful and timid. The condition is characterized by dread of the future, involuntary quivering, trembling, and feeling distressed and suddenly upset.

Yawning - Involuntary opening of the mouth with deep inhalation of air.

REPRODUCTIVE FEMALE

Breast Neoplasm - A tumor or cancer, of either of the two milk-secreting organs on the chest of a woman.

Menorrhagia - Abnormally heavy menstrual period or a menstrual flow that has continued for an unusually long period of time.

Menstrual Cramps - Painful, involuntary uterus contractions that women experience around the time of their menstrual period, sometimes causing pain in the lower back and thighs.

Menstrual Disorder - A disturbance or derangement in the normal function of a woman's menstrual period.

Pelvic Inflammation - The reaction of the body to infectious, allergic or chemical irritation, which, in turn, causes tissue irritation, injury, or bacterial infection characterized by pain, redness, swelling, and sometimes loss of function. The reaction usually begins in the uterus and spreads to the fallopian tubes, ovaries and other areas in the hipbone region of the body.

Premenstrual Syndrome - Various physical and mental symptoms commonly experienced by women of childbearing age usually 2 to 7 days before the start of their monthly period. There are over 150 symptoms including eating binges, behavioral changes, moodiness, irritability, fatigue, fluid retention, breast tenderness, headaches, bloating, anxiety and depression. The symptoms cease shortly after the period begins and disappear with menopause.

Spotting Between Menses - Abnormal bleeding between periods. Unusual spotting between menstrual cycles.

RESPIRATORY SYSTEM

Asthma - A disease of the breathing system initiated by an allergic reaction or a chemical, with repeated attacks of coughing, sticky mucus, wheezing, shortness of breath and a tight feeling in the chest. The disease can reach a state where it stops a person from exhaling, leading to unconsciousness and death.

Breath Shortness - Unnatural breathing, using a lot of effort resulting in not enough air taken in by the body.

Bronchitis - Inflammation of the two main breathing tubes leading from the windpipe to the lungs. The disease is marked by coughing, a low-grade fever, chest pain and hoarseness. Can also be caused by an allergic reaction.

Coughing - A cough is the response to an irritation, such as mucus, that causes the muscles controlling the breathing process to expel air from the lungs suddenly and noisily to keep the air passages free from the irritating material.

Laryngitis - Inflammation of the voice box characterized by hoarseness, sore throat, and coughing. It can be caused by straining the voice or exposure to infectious, allergic or chemical irritation.

Nasal Congestion - The presence of an abnormal amount of fluid.

Pneumonia Tracheitis - Bacterial infection of the air passageways and lungs that causes redness, swelling and pain in the windpipe. Other symptoms are high fever, chills, pain in the chest, difficulty breathing and coughing with mucus discharge.

Rhinitis - Chemical irritation causing pain, redness and swelling in the mucus membranes of the nose.

Sinus Congestion - The mucus-lined areas of the bones in the face that are thought to help warm and moisten air to the nose. These areas become clogged with excess fluid or become infected.

Sinus Headache - An abnormal amount of fluid in the hollows of the facial bone structure, especially around the nose. This excess fluid creates pressure, causing pain in the head.

Sinusitis - The body reacting to chemical irritation causing redness, swelling and pain in the area of the hollows in the facial bones especially around the nose.

SKELETAL

Neck/Shoulder Pain - Hurtful sensations of the nerve endings caused by damage to the tissues in the neck and shoulder, signaling danger of disease.

SKIN AND APPENDAGES (SKIN, LEGS AND ARMS)

Acne - Eruptions of the oil glands of the skin, especially on the face, marked by pimples, blackheads, whiteheads, bumps and more severely, by cysts and scarring.

Alopecia - The loss of hair, baldness.

Angioedema - Intense itching and swelling welts on the skin called hives caused by an allergic reaction to internal or external agents. The reaction is common to a food or a drug. Chronic cases can last for a long period of time.

Dermatitis - Generally irritated skin that can be caused by any of a number of irritating conditions, such as parasites, fungus, bacteria, or foreign substances causing an allergic reaction. It is a general inflammation of the skin.

Dry Lips - The lack of normal moisture in the fleshy folds that surround the mouth.

Dry Skin - The lack of normal moisture/oils in the surface layer of the body. The skin is the body's largest organ.

Epidermal Necrolysis - An abnormal condition in which a large portion of the skin becomes intensely red and peels off like a second-degree burn. Symptoms often include blistering.

Eczema - A severe or continuing skin disease marked by redness, crusting and scaling, with watery blisters and itching. It is often difficult to treat and will sometimes go away only to reappear again.

Folliculitis - Inflammation of a follicle (small body sac), especially a hair follicle. A hair follicle contains the root of a hair.

Furunculosis - Skin boils that show up repeatedly.

Lipoma - A tumor of mostly fat cells that is not health endangering.

Pruritus - Extreme itching of often-undamaged skin.

Rash - A skin eruption or discoloration that may or may not be itching, tingling, burning or painful. It may be caused by an allergy, a skin irritation or a skin disease.

Skin Nodule - A bulge, knob, swelling or outgrowth in the skin that is a mass of tissue or cells.

RELATED TO THE SENSES

Conjunctivitis - Infection of the membrane that covers the eyeball and lines the eyelid, caused by a virus, allergic reaction or an irritating chemical. It is characterized by redness, a discharge of fluid and itching.

Dry Eyes - Not enough moisture in the eyes.

Earache - Pain in the ear.

Eye Infection - The invasion of the eye tissue by a bacteria, virus, fungus, etc, causing damage to the tissue, with toxicity. Infection spreading in the body progresses into disease.

Eye Irritation - An inflammation of the eye.

Metallic Taste - A range of taste impairment from distorted taste to a complete loss of taste.

Pupils Dilated - Abnormal expansion of the black circular opening in the center of the eye.

Taste Alteration - Abnormal flavor detection in food.

Tinnitus - A buzzing, ringing or whistling sound in one or both ears occurring from the use of certain drugs.

Vision Abnormal - Normal images are seen differently by the viewer than by others.

Vision Blurred - Eyesight is dim or indistinct and hazy in outline or appearance.

Visual Disturbance - Eyesight is interfered with or interrupted. Examples of disturbances are light sensitivity and the inability to easily distinguish colors.

URINARY SYSTEM

Blood in Urine - Blood is present when one empties the liquid waste product of the kidneys through the bladder by urinating in the toilet, turning the water pink to bright red. Or spots of blood are observable in the water after urinating.

Dysuria - Difficult or painful urination.

Kidney Stone - Small hard masses of salt deposits that the kidney forms.

Urinary Frequency - Having to urinate more often than usual or between unusually short time periods.

Urinary Tract Infection - An invasion of bacteria, viruses, fungi, etc., of the system in the body. This starts with the kidneys, which eliminate urine from the body. If the invasion goes unchecked, it can injure tissue and progress into disease.

Urinary Urgency - A sudden compelling urge to urinate, accompanied by discomfort in the bladder.

UROGENITAL (URINARY TR ACT)

Anorgasmia - Failure to experience an orgasm.

Ejaculation Disorder- Dysfunction during orgasm.

Menstrual Disorder - Dysfunction of the discharge during the monthly menstrual cycle.

VIOLENT OR PHYSICALLY DANGEROUS SIDE EFFECTS

Acute Renal Failure - The kidneys stop excreting waste products properly, leading to rapid poisoning (toxicity) in the body.

Anaphylaxis - A violent, sudden, and severe drop in blood pressure caused by a re-exposure to a foreign protein or a second dosage of a drug that may be fatal unless emergency treatment is given right away.

Grand Mal Seizures (or Convulsions) - A recurring sudden, violent and involuntary attack of muscle spasms with a loss of consciousness.

Neuroleptic Malignant Syndrome - A life threatening, rare reaction to an anti-psychotic drug marked by fever, muscular rigidity, changed mental status and dysfunction of the autonomic nervous system.

Pancreatitis - Chemical irritation with redness, swelling and pain in the pancreas where digestive enzymes and hormones are secreted.

QT Prolongation - A very fast heart rhythm disturbance that is too fast for the heart to beat effectively so the blood to the brain falls, causing a sudden loss of consciousness. May cause sudden cardiac arrest.

Rhabdomyolysis - The breakdown and release of muscle fibers into the circulatory system.

Serotonin Syndrome - A disorder brought on by excessive levels of serotonin. Symptoms include euphoria, drowsiness, sustained and rapid eye movement, agitation, reflexes overreacting, rapid muscle contractions, abnormal movements of the foot, clumsiness, feeling drunk and dizzy without any intake of alcohol, jaw muscles contracting and relaxing excessively, muscle twitching, high body temperature, rigid body, rotating mental status - including

confusion and excessive happiness - diarrhea and loss of consciousness.

Thrombocytopenia - An abnormal decrease in the number of blood platelets in the circulatory system. A decrease in platelets causes a decrease in the ability of the blood to clot when necessary.

Torsades de Pointes - Unusually rapid heart rhythm starting in the lower heart chambers. If the short bursts of rapid heart rhythm continue for a prolonged period, it can degenerate into a more rapid rhythm and can be fatal.

Benzodiazepine Side Effects

CARDIAC DISORDERS

Palpitation - Perceptible forcible pulsation of the heart, usually with an increase in frequency or force, with or without irregularity in rhythm.

Tachycardia - Rapid heart rate.

EAR AND LABYRINTH DISORDERS

Ear pain - Any pain connected to the inner or outer portion of the ear.

Tinnitus - A sound in one ear or both ears; buzzing, ringing, or whistling, occurring without an external stimulus and usually caused by a separate condition.

49

Vertigo - A sensation of irregular or whirling motion, either of oneself or of external objects.

EYE DISORDER

Blurred vision - Compared to normal, a distortion of vision.

Mydriasis - Prolonged abnormal dilation of the pupil of the eye induced by a drug or caused by disease.

Photophobia - An abnormal sensitivity to or intolerance of light, especially by the eyes, as may be caused by eye inflammation. An abnormal fear of light.

GASTROINTESTIONAL DISORDERS

Abdominal pain - Pain between the chest and pelvis, stomach, intestines, liver, spleen, and pancreas.

Constipation - Difficulty having normal bowel movement.

Diarrhea - Excessive and frequent evacuation of watery feces.

Dry mouth - When the mouth is dry beyond what might be normal.

Dyspepsia - Disturbed digestion; indigestion.

Dysphagia - Difficulty in swallowing or inability to swallow.

Nausea - A feeling of sickness with the urge to vomit.

Pharyngolaryngeal syndrome - Of or pertaining to the larynx or pharynx.

Salivary hypersecretion - A continual or excessive

amount of saliva.

Vomiting - Ejecting all or part of the stomach contents.

GENERAL DISORDERS

Asthenia - Loss or lack of bodily strength.

Chest tightness - A feeling in the chest of contraction.

Edema - An accumulation of an excessive amount of watery fluid in cells, tissues, or body cavities.

Fatigue – The body feeling drained of energy

Feeling drunk - Feelings associated with drinking too much alcohol.

Feeling hot or cold - An uncontrollable feeling of being too hot or cold that is abnormal for the temperature.

Feeling jittery - An uneasy feeling often associated with the inability to remain still.

Hangover - Feeling like the day after consuming too much alcohol. All or a few hangover sensations may be present.

Increased energy - An abnormal amount of energy.

Loss of control of legs – Inability to control legs.

Malaise - A vague feeling of bodily discomfort.

Pyrexia – Fever

Rigors - Shivering or trembling, as caused by a chill. A state of rigidity in living tissues or organs that prevents response to stimuli.

Sluggishness - A fatigue type feeling or dull.

Thirst - An abnormal sensation of needing liquid.

Weakness - A reduced state of normal energy and stamina.

INFECTIONS AND INFESTATIONS

Influenza symptoms - The body feeling and at times the manifestation of flue like symptoms.

Upper respiratory tract infections - Infection of the nose, sinuses, pharynx (part of neck and throat) or larynx (commonly known as the voice box).

MENTAL DISORDERS

Abnormal dreams - Nightmares or dreams that are upsetting to the individual.

Aggression - Hostile or destructive behavior or actions.

Agitation - A feeling where something or anything could set a person toward anger or combativeness.

Anger - Uncontrollable and volatile emotion with rage; usually an attempt to stop someone or something.

Anxiety - A state of uneasiness and apprehension, as about future uncertainties. A state of intense apprehension, uncertainty, and fear resulting from the anticipation of a threatening event or situation, often to a degree that normal physical and psychological functioning is disrupted.

Apathy - A feeling of no hope, such as if anything can be done it would not work.

Bradyphrenia - A slowness of the mind.

Confusion - An impaired orientation with respect to time, place or the form of an event.

Depersonalization - A state in which the normal sense of personal identity and reality is lost, characterized by feelings that one's actions and speech cannot be controlled.

Depressed mood - A lowering of the state of mind or emotion compared to what a person normally feels.

Depression - A feeling of no hope.

Derealization - The feeling that things in one's surroundings are strange, unreal, or somehow altered, as seen in schizophrenia.

Disorientation – A loss of sense of direction, position, or relationship with one's surroundings. A temporary or permanent state of confusion regarding place, time or personal identity.

Dysphonia - An emotional state marked by anxiety, depression, and restlessness.

Euphoric mood - A feeling of great happiness or well-being, commonly exaggerated and not necessarily well founded.

Hallucination - False or distorted perception of objects or events with a compelling sense of their reality, usually resulting from a traumatic life event or drugs.

Homicidal ideation - The formation of the idea or having the mental image of murder.

Hypomania - A mild form of mania, characterized by hyperactivity and euphoria.

Impulse control - A sudden pushing or driving force. A sudden wish or urge that prompts an unpremeditated act or feeling; an abrupt inclination.

Insomnia - Chronic inability to fall asleep or remain asleep for an adequate length of time.

Irritability - 1. The capacity to respond to stimuli. 2. Abnormal or excessive sensitivity to stimuli of organism, organ, or body part.

Libido decreased - Sexual desire decreased

Libido increased - Sexual desire increased.

Logorrhea - Incoherent talkativeness.

Mania - A manifestation of bipolar disorder characterized by profuse and rapidly changing ideas, exaggerated gaiety, and excessive physical activity.

Mood swings - The up and or down movement of emotions that are uncontrollable.

Nervousness - Easily agitated or distressed.

Nightmare - A dream creating intense fear, horror, and distress.

Psychomotor retardation - The retardation of movement and or mental process.

Restlessness - An uneasy feeling of not being able to be where one is located comfortably.

Suicidal ideation - The formation of an idea or mental image of killing one self.

METABOLISM AND NUTRITION DISORDERS

Anorexia - Loss of appetite, usually including a fear of becoming obese or an aversion toward food.

Appetite decreased - A decrease in the feeling one needs food for survival.

Appetite increased - An increase of the desire for food for survival.

MUSCULOSKELETAL AND CONNECTIVE TISSUE DISORDERS

Arthralgia - Severe pain in a joint.

Back pain - An unexplained pain anywhere in the back.

Muscle cramps - Muscle being contracted to the point of discomfort.

Muscle twitching - A rhythmic or irregular involuntary movement of any muscle.

Myalgia - Muscular pain or tenderness, especially when nonspecific.

Pain in limb - Pain in arm or leg.

NERVOUS SYSTEM DISORDERS

Amnesia - The loss or impairment of memory.

Ataxia - Loss of the ability to coordinate muscular movement.

Coordination abnormal - Maintaining balance of the body difficult in comparison to what is normal for the person.

Disturbance in attention - Not able to remain as focused as one was able to in the past.

Dizziness - A disorienting sensation such as faintness, light-headedness, or unsteadiness.

Dysarthria - Difficulty in articulating words due to emotional stress or to paralysis or incoordination of the muscles used in speaking.

Dyskinesia - An impairment in the ability to control movements, characterized by spasmodic or repetitive motions of lack of coordination.

Headache - A continual or time specific duration with pressure or pain within the head.

Hypersomnia - A condition in which one sleeps for an excessively long time but is normal in the waking intervals.

Hypoesthesia - Drowsiness.

Hypotonia - Reduced tension or pressure, as of the intraocular fluid in the eyeball.

Memory impairment - Not able to recall an instance from the past as well as before.

Mental impairment - The ability to think and reason diminished.

Paresthesia - A skin sensation, such as burning, prickling, itching.

Sedation - An over expression of reduction of anxiety, stress, irritability or excitement.

Seizures - A sudden attack, spasm, or convulsion, as in epilepsy.

Sleep apnea – A temporary cessation of breathing while asleep.

Sleep talking - Speaking words while asleep.

Somnolence - A state of drowsiness; sleepiness. A condition of semi- consciousness approaching coma.

Stupor - A state of impaired consciousness characterized by a marked diminution in the capacity to react to environmental stimuli.

Syncope - A brief loss of consciousness caused by a sudden fall of blood pressure or failure of cardiac systole, resulting in cerebral anemia.

Tremor - An involuntary trembling movement.

RENAL, THORACIC, AND MEDIASTINAL DISORDERS

Difficulty in micturition - Difficulty with urination or the frequency of.

Urinary frequency - An abnormal frequency of urination.

Urinary incontinence - Involuntary leakage of urine.

REPRODUCTIVE SYSTEM AND BRE AST DISORDERS

Dysmenorrhea - A condition marked by painful menstruation.

Premenstrual syndrome - A group of symptoms, including abdominal bloating, breast tenderness, headache, fatigue, irritability, and depression.

Sexual dysfunction - A non-normal, for the individual, behavior or ability to have sex.

RESPIRATORY, THORACIC AND MEDIASTINAL DISORDERS

Choking sensation - A feeling of choking with or without cause.

Dyspnea - Difficulty in breathing, often associated with lung or heart disease and resulting in shortness of breath.

Epistaxis - Nosebleed.

Hyperventilation - Abnormally fast or deep respiration resulting in the loss of carbon dioxide from the blood, thereby causing a decrease in blood pressure and sometimes fainting.

Nasal congestion - A stoppage or restriction of the nasal passage.

Rhinitis - Inflammation of the nasal membranes.

Rhinorrhea - A discharge from the mucous membrane, especially if excessive.

VASCULAR DISORDERS

Hot flashes – A sudden, brief sensation of heat, often over the entire body, caused by a transient dilation of blood vessels of the skin.

Hypotension - Abnormally low arterial blood pressure.

SKIN AND SUBCUTANEOUS TISSUE DISORDERS

Clamminess - Abnormally moist, sticky and cold to the touch.

Pruritus - Severe itching, often of undamaged skin.

Rash - A skin eruption.

Sweating increased - Abnormal increase of perspiration.

Urticaria - A skin condition characterized by welts that itch intensely, caused by an allergic reaction, an infection, or nervous condition.

Chapter 5

Things To Be
Aware Of

THERE ARE SEVERAL medical situations you need to be aware of before you start this program. First let me repeat, check with your doctor before starting this program. Medically and physically, do this for your health and safety as you travel through this process.

I understand there could be a problem: possibly your doctor does not support tapering off the medication.

This is your journey. Find those who will help you travel the proven successful road laid out for you.

Physical Conditions and Drug Interactions

Many people have contacted me over the years, asking about their activities and/or medications taken and whether they can use these in combination with The Road Back Program. My answer? Check with your doctor about medications and how these could interact with other supplements, vitamins, drugs and so on. Having said that, I know various medical conditions and/or drugs could possibly interfere with this program, including the following:

1. Blood thinners and heart medication

Omega 3 and vitamin E both thin the blood. Taking either of these supplements, in conjunction with a medication that is already thinning your blood, could be contra-indicated, or not advised. If your blood pressure is too low or too high and you are taking medication in an attempt to correct that condition, you need to closely monitor your blood pressure.

2. Clotting agents

The JNK Capsules used in The Road Back Program contain vitamin K. If you are on medication for your heart get with your physician before starting this program.

3. Diabetes Medication

If you are diabetic and taking medication to raise or lower glucose levels, when using this program you need to monitor your glucose levels closely. The JNK Capsules, will probably bring your glucose levels back to a normal range quickly and if you are taking medication to lower your glucose level you will find the need for a piece of fruit quickly in order to get your glucose level up again.

The problem is the drug you are taking, not the supplement.

The supplements work dramatically and quickly to balance out our bodily functions.

Alternative Therapies

While I have personally seen the results from natural health and healing practices, each has its own purpose and end result. Additionally, I have found they can too often be counter-productive when used in conjunction with The Road Back Program. Any alternative therapy or health practice that recommends additional nutrients, supplements, vitamins, drips, sprays, drinks and methodologies can and do exacerbate, aggravate or make worse, the very sensitive process we are trying to guide you through now.

Due to your drugs, your system is essentially balanced on the "head of a pin," meaning that your tolerance for anything can be, or is, very limited.

The Road Back Program has been researched and developed around very specific parameters, undercutting any other health products. While these other health products might be great in a healthy, balanced body, they often do not mix well with psychiatric medications and your tapering process. Right now, you need to slowly and safely taper off your drug. Add other health products back into your daily regime after you have completed this venture. Once completely and safely off the drug, by all means, help yourself.

While on The Road Back Program, taking various health products adds one more thing to an already overloaded system. Therefore, I emphatically recommend you evaluate these alternative therapies, practices, nutritional items and restrict them until successfully completing your program. Specifically, anything that moves medications too rapidly or inhibits their metabolism through your body should be avoided.

Chapter 6

General
Pre -Taper And Taper
Instructions

DESPITE APPARENT REDUNDANCY, what I am about to say cannot be said too many times, so bear with me.

As you start your road back, I want your journey to be as successful and as smooth as possible. Therefore, I repeat: you cannot simply quit your prescription medications cold turkey. The illegal use of prescription drugs are the most abused drugs by young adults and teens at this time, and that may present a little difficulty with tapering off of psychoactive medications slowly for you, if you are using the drug without a prescription. You still need to taper the drugs to help prevent the psychotic episodes associated with an abrupt withdrawal. Go to the chapter of this book that details how to reduce the medication and follow the instructions as closely as possible.

You must methodically taper off most drugs, giving your body all possible assistance to ensure you fully complete this program and are not driven back onto your drug.

Your program consists of a two-part process: First, the pre-taper, which is usually done in one week. If you need more time on the pre-taper go-ahead and spend the time, but the final relief may not come until you are reducing the drug or until you are completely off the drug.

This is a journey back to you through steady steps that become more and more certain over time.

Once finished with the pre-taper, you will start the actual taper. You will start to reduce the drug while continuing your supplements. The number of drugs you are currently taking, and your speed of progress each step along the way, will determine the length of the tapering process.

This chapter is an overview of the pre-tapering and tapering process, and what you will do no matter which drug or drugs you are taking.

These steps are vitally important to your success. Please study them carefully to ensure confidence when beginning your personal program.

The Purpose of the Pre-Taper

Just as in running a marathon, swimming a mile, buying a house, or having a baby, you have to build up to the ultimate goal. The same applies with The Road Back Program. You need to stretch your muscles, get some correct nutrients into your system and know how your daily schedule will change. The Pre Taper will set you up for a smooth reduction off your medications.

The Pre-Taper Goals

Elimination, or a *drastic* reduction, of all existing side effects caused by the drug.

Determining which supplements created the positive change.

When you know the exact supplement that eliminated the side effects, you will know how to eliminate that side effect, if it recurs during the drug reduction phase of your program.

The reasoning: If a withdrawal side effect begins during the taper, odds are high that it was one of the existing side effects you had *before you started your pre-taper.*

An example of the importance of the pre-taper is found in the Introduction to *The Art of War* by Sun Tzu, from Thomas Cleary's translation.

"Plan for what is difficult while it is easy, do what is great while it is small. The most difficult things in the world must be done while they are still easy; the greatest things in the world must be done while they are still small."

Nutritional Supplements

Review the Chapter "Nutritionals Used on The Road Back Program" and make sure you have the nutritional supplements on hand. The day before you start your pre-taper, review which supplements you will be taking the next day, and the times you will be taking them. If you will be carrying the supplements with you during the day, and need to put those quantities into smaller containers, do so. If you know that you have a busy schedule on the day that you will start, or any day following that, prepare by making a note of when you need to take your supplements and how you can arrange to do so. If you do not usually carry water with you, or have it available where you will be, take some with you.

Today, with this program a person can taper completely off their drug quickly. The changes to the program are fewer supplements used and a two third reduction in time that it takes to complete the entire program. The pre- taper has been able to change from taking twenty-two days to seven days.

Your Daily Journal:

Every day you will keep a written record of your progress in a journal.

You are free to copy the journal found in the next chapter and put together your own, or you can find pre-made journals at The Road Back website. In your Daily Journal you will note certain information over the course of a 24-hour period. These specific statistics are important because they will help you find your way back to center, if you falter at any point during the program. Before going to bed each night, or during the day as you take each step, write down the following:

- The date.

- The time of all medications you took that day and dosage amount.

- All food and drinks, including coffee, water, alcohol, etc; times you ate or drank, and the amount.

- Rate your own progress as to how you feel.

- Rate your energy, appetite, mood and exercise.

- Include anything that you added or deleted from your

daily routine.

Keeping the journal allows you to review changes and determine which changes made positive improvements. However, if a problem occurs, the journal allows you to look back and locate which change may have made a negative impact. Locating such change will enable you to quickly fix what happened and get yourself back on track.

For example, you may have increased your supplements too quickly or too much, and now you need to reduce them to the quantity you were taking when you last felt good. Or possibly you felt so good from the pre-taper that you added exercise into your day, which created a negative change. Whatever the case, it could be a small and seemingly insignificant change, or it could be a major change that you did not realize you had made. Using your Daily Journal, you will be able to find your way back. The Daily Journal will act like a positive voice sitting on your shoulder reminding you of what works for you, and what does not.

By noting the exact quantity of each supplement you have taken daily, you will know the positive changes are a direct result of the exact amounts and times you took your supplements.

Graph Your Success

Along the way it will also help if you were to keep a daily graph. Sometimes it can be easy to lose track of where you actually started from, but with a daily graph, it is easy to look back and see where you have been and more importantly, to look at the current trend you are having. The example graphs on the following page are quite common:

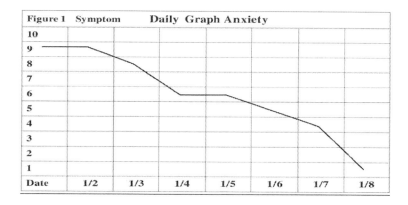

Figure 1 shows a person starting the pre-taper with an anxiety rating of 9 on day 1. At the end of day 3 of the pre-taper the anxiety drops to an 8 and at the end of day 4 the anxiety level is now down to a 6 rating.

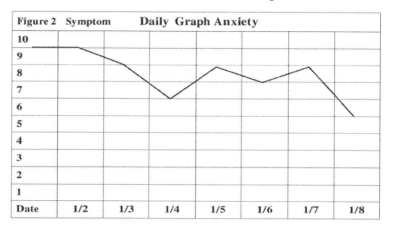

Your individual graph may even look like the chart of Figure 2

Figure 2 is not a constant and steady decline of anxiety, but while you study the graph you will be able to see the overall trend changing and the anxiety level decreasing. As you leave the world of drug induced anxiety, you enter back into what is normal or the all too common levels of anxiety. The common is; none of us have a continual steady line without any anxiety or anxiousness. As we cope with daily events of life our anxiety may go up and down several times each day. The Road Back Program will be offering an anxiety solution program in the near future to help individuals learn how to handle the daily common and normal anxiety.

You could place fatigue, depression or any other condition in the Figure 1 and Figure 2 graphs. Please do that. If depression is your main symptom and not anxiety, graph the depression, if it is fatigue, graph fatigue etc.

Take your graphs in to your physician and show your physician the changes you are now experiencing. This will help your physician see an objective piece instead of a purely subjective of "how you feel".

Deviation from The Road Back Program

You might think deviating from the program would be obvious and easy to detect. Not always.

The Road Back Program usually works quickly, with the person experiencing a vast improvement within the first few days. This blessing can also be a curse. In the first years of the program, a person would typically feel a major positive change about halfway through the tapering portion and start doing things they have put off for years, such as exercise, dieting. Now they frequently experience major positive change after a few days on the pre-taper

69

and have the urge to introduce new things to their daily life. The creation of the supplements and the time of day each is taken have greatly sped up the program. Imagine feeling as though you had never taken a drug only one week after starting the pre-taper part of The Road Back Program.

However, when this major positive change occurs, a person can feel so good that he or she begins doing things they have wanted to do for years, such as quitting smoking, giving up coffee or starting a major exercise program.

Then they suddenly crash and wonder why

I first experienced this curse in 1999 when a woman called who was tapering off her medication. After first doing well, suddenly she was not. She had tried to taper off an antidepressant medication several times over the years before starting The Road Back Program, never reducing the drug without extreme withdrawal and always returning to her original dosage. This time she had been halfway off her medication and feeling great.

It took two weeks to figure out what changed. I asked every question I could think of; there was something she was doing differently. I finally found out that typically, every six months, she went onto an all-protein diet. This was so "normal" for her she never thought to mention, or view it, as a major change in her lifestyle. However, this diet change hugely impacted her progress, and was the major deviation from the program. Once the change was discovered, she re-started her tapering program from square one and successfully completed tapering off the antidepressant.

I cannot over stress looking for and finding obvious as well as subtle changes if you experience a negative change during this program.

Another major deviation from the program can occur – you feel so good, you forget to take your medication(s). This is a no-no, but happens. Lower the medication only at specific amounts and make that gradual reduction. Numerous people over the years have begun a pre-taper while suffering from widely varying side effects. Taking psychiatric medications for years, they had tried to get off the drugs countless times. After beginning the pre-taper and finally sleeping through the night for the first time in months, their daytime anxiety vanished. Three days later, they forgot to take their medication at bedtime. The next day, they went into full withdrawal and began to question whether The Road Back Program was right for them. The only problem was forgetting to take their medication.

These variations or deviations from the program can also be extremely troubling for a doctor. He or she can only help guide you through the steps with all the information on hand. Again, it is imperative that: a) you write everything down in your Daily Journal, including things you might think have no bearing whatsoever, and b) bring your Daily Journal to your doctor visits, so that together you can chart your progress and get back to square one if needed.

Major Improvement

A major improvement is what you are going for with the pre-taper.

If you have extreme daytime anxiety and are able to reduce it to a point where you have to stop and look for anxiety to even see or feel any, you have had a major improvement.

If you could not sleep more than two hours a night and are now able to sleep four to five hours, wake up and then go back to sleep, that is a major improvement.

If every joint in your body ached, and now you have only a little ache in the morning when you awake that goes away within the first few minutes, you have experienced a major improvement.

If you felt a major depression every day and now you feel a little depressed occasionally, you have had a major improvement.

If you feel like you are not even taking a medication now, you have had a major improvement.

Major changes are what you are going for during the pre-taper. The goal is to alleviate major complaints or reduce them to the point of being very acceptable and not in the way of day-to-day life, so that you can fully taper off the medication and "live life."

Steady State: The term "steady state" has special definitions in biochemistry, chemistry, electronics and even macroeconomics.

In The Road Back Program "steady state" is defined as: A constant level or a level of action that allows a balance between two or more substances.

A *constant level* would be maintaining a level of a supplement in the body to a degree where it never drops below a certain point. Much like the half- life of medication, keeping enough of a substance in the body at a specific strength gives a result. If you skip a dosage of medication, withdrawal begins. If you skip a serving of a supplement, withdrawal does not take place, but you do lose the steady or constant state of the supplement.

A level of action that allows a balance between two or more substances is different from a *constant level.* Psychiatric medications alter hormones and the adrenals. When a "steady state" occurs with the nutritionals at a *constant level,* the cells will use the nutrients to begin working with each other, balancing each other, allowing the cells to receive energy and exchange back to other cells desired substances for optimum survival.

During the pre-taper, one goal is finding the "steady state" of each nutritional for your body. Age, height, weight, gender, how long you have been using a medication or the type of medication you might be using cannot be used to predict the correct amount of a nutritional in this program. This takes trial and success.

If You Have Anxiety, Insomnia, Fatigue, What to Expect

You can and should expect a rapid reduction in anxiety, insomnia or fatigue. The JNK Capsules, Adrenalpin, and Neuro Endure Mini work fast with these conditions. With the addition of the Body Calm Daytime Relief and Body Calm Supreme, the anxiety and insomnia should now be a thing of the past.

Calcium-Induced Side Effects

If you have anxiety or insomnia and are taking a calcium supplement, please read this section carefully. In 2005, we found one common factor of anxiety with people taking anti-anxiety drugs and that common factor was the use of calcium. Once they stopped the calcium supplement their anxiety and insomnia improved greatly. This was later found to be the case for people taking all types of medication, not just antianxiety medication. In time we also found the calcium/anxiety problem to exist for those not even taking a psychoactive medication.

Calcium Solution Breakthrough

After 6 years of research we have found a person can take calcium, however it needs to be calcium citrate with the right ratio and type of magnesium along with a combination of vitamin C, vitamin D and another supplement called NAC. You will read a bit in this book about the gene called JNK and the calcium formula we recommend also works on stopping the over activation of one part of the JNK gene.

Calcium stimulates electrical discharge of the nerves. The stimulation of nerve impulses is one problem associated with the incorrect calcium. If you need to take calcium daily or if you have agitation, daytime anxiety or insomnia, use the calcium citrate.

Calcium-induced side effects can include:

- Hyperkinesia: an abnormal increase in muscular activity, hyperactivity, especially in children.

- Hyperthermia: unusually high body temperature. Hyper aggression.

- Audiogenic seizures: Seizures caused by loud sounds and noises.

- Reaction to bright light or a reaction to a sudden increase of light. Increased anxiety.

74

- Psychosis.

- Numbness around the mouth. Tingling in the extremities. Shortness of breath.

  Your Next Step – Make a copy of the Daily Journal found in the next chapter and then make yourself some graphs found in the following chapter, then proceed to the chapter matching the drug/s you wish to taper. If you are tapering from more than one drug, make sure to read all of the drug chapters that relate to your situation.

Chapter 7

Daily Journal

Date:_____Pre-Taper/Taper (Circle One) Day #___ Step#___

Note: Do not change eating or exercise habits during this program

Current Drugs & Dosages: (List all taken, time of day and amount)

_____ _____ _____ _____
_____ _____ _____ _____

Food and Liquid:

(List all food and liquid consumed, time of day and amount)

The Road Back Nutritionals: (List all taken, time of day and amount)

Rate the Following Areas Using a Scale of 1 to 10 : (Rate daytime anxiety at bedtime and rate the previous night's sleep first thing in the morning. Rate all other items before bedtime. Rate with the #1 being the best and use #10 as the worst)

Symptom	1-10 Rating	List All Changes Made During the Day
Aches		
Anxiety		
Appetite		
Body Pains		
Energy		
Exercise		
Fatigue		
Mood		
Sleep		

Chapter 8

Graph Your Success

A GRAPH FOR each symptom you are rating each day can greatly help track your progress and allow you to look back at how far you have come.

See an example below of how to fill in the graph. The next page is a blank graph for you to copy or recreate on your own.

Pre-Taper / Taper (Circle one)   Day # _____ Rate with the #1 being the best and use #10 as the worst.

Symptom	Anxiety						
10							
9							
8							
7							
6							
5							
4							
3							
2							
1							
Date	1/2	1/3	1/4	1/5	1/6	1/7	1/8

Notice the trend changes in the graph. After three days a level period starts for two days and then changes again. Look at the long term trend of your graphs to determine improvement.

This is a normal daily trend during the beginning of the pre-taper. If you have already quit taking the medication and are suffering from withdrawal side effects, make sure you use these graphs. I understand you need hope, and seeing for yourself may spark the hope that inspires you to continue and make it back.

After graphing each day and symptom for a period of time, you will see a longer-term trend. Placing each graph side-by-side you can easily see your ratings for several weeks and your trend for each symptom.

Make sure you take your Daily Journal and graphs to your doctor visits.

By running each graph for seven days, you can attach one completed graph to seven days of your Daily Journal and create a weekly file.

Chapter 9

Anti-Anxiety, Anticonvulsants, Benzodiazepine, And Sleep Medication Pre-Taper

Starting Your Pre-Taper

Note: This pre-taper addresses several types of medication, as indicated in the chapter title. For the rest of this chapter, the word "benzodiazepine" is used alone to encompass all of the medications included in the chapter title (Benzodiazepine, Antianxiety, Anticonvulsant and Sleep Medication).

During the pre-taper and taper, you will address the immune system–the hypothalamic pituitary adrenal-axis, cortisol and the adrenals, along with enzymes that regulate anxiety, sleep and other symptoms resulting from benzodiazepine usage. While many of these symptoms may be viewed as mental (anxiety, insomnia, and other subjective symptoms), we will address them as physical symptoms.

You may already have heart palpitations or aches and pains throughout the body. These side effects are addressed with this program as well as any and all side effects, you may be experiencing.

You will begin your pre-taper by taking the Neuro Endure Mini, JNK Capsules, Body Calm Daytime Relief and Body Calm Supreme With Melatonin or you can use Body Calm Supreme Melatonin Free. These are the basic supplements used for a benzodiazepine taper, and the majority of you will not need any other supplements.

If you are also taking an antidepressant, you should reduce the benzodiazepine first. You will be taking; Neuro Endure Mini, JNK Capsules, Body Calm Daytime Relief and Body Calm Supreme.

These supplements should take care of most or all daytime anxiety, panic attacks, sleep problems etc. If you have taken a benzodiazepine for a prolonged period and have depression or a tingling or numbness of the extremities, the JNK Capsules will be vital. Prolonged use of a benzodiazepine massively depletes the B vitamin biotin and leads to depression and tingling or numbness of an extremity. To help address this, the JNK Capsules includes biotin in the formula.

A few individuals will also have fatigue during the daytime while taking these medications. If you are one of them, handle the daytime anxiety first, have 3 good nights of sleep in succession and re-evaluate the fatigue. For most people it will go away with 3 good nights of sleep. If the fatigue is still present you can increase the Neuro Endure Mini by 1 tablet to help lift the fatigue.

Remember, as soon as you start the pre-taper, you simultaneously begin keeping your Daily Journal and keeping your graphs up to date.

Make sure to note in your journal when existing side effects stop or when there is a major improvement. This is very important.

Anxiety first thing in the morning and again in the afternoon is a very common side effect of benzodiazepines. By the time you are ready to go to sleep at night, you are too stressed out and fatigued from dealing with anxiety difficulties all day long that sleep simply may not come. You could easily end up feeling depressed due to this endless cycle of anxiety, insomnia, anxiety, and insomnia. **Take the Adrenalpin as well if this applies to you.**

Part of the process of handling sleep is by addressing the anxiety that is usually present during the daytime. You will be taking the Body Calm Daytime Relief during the daytime to help with anxiety, which will also help set you up for a good night's sleep when it is bedtime. It is much easier to go to sleep if you are not all ramped up from daily activities or constant daily anxiety.

If you are also experiencing some degree of depression, do not be surprised if the depression lifts during the pre-taper as your ability to sleep improves, daytime anxiety abates or other symptoms you may be experiencing vanish. Even so, as you start to experience relief from your symptoms, *do not change anything*; just continue with the program. There are still many, many gains available as you continue through and complete The Road Back Program.

There are optional supplements you can use along the way, but they are here for specific symptoms that not everyone will have. Again, most people will do very well with only taking the Neuro Endure Mini, JNK Capsules, Body Calm Daytime Relief and Body Calm

Supreme.

If you would like to include some optional supplements, read through the chapter "Nutritionals Used on The Road Back Program" for a full list of optional supplements.

If mood is a constant problem for you, try out a bottle of Omega 3 Supreme TG. Put 3 of the softgels in your mouth and bite through the softgel, swallow the oil and remove the softgels from your mouth. If this is what you needed for mood you will feel the difference in minutes.

What to do next:

1. Read through the chapter How to Taper Anti-anxiety, Anticonvulsants, Benzodiazepines and Sleep Medication.

2. Consult with your prescribing physician and/or pharmacist and layout your drug taper schedule.

3. Plan out the second and third reduction of the medication as well at this point to ensure you are ready with the correct dosages of the drug.

The Pre-Taper

For the next 7 days you will be doing your pre-taper. You do not reduce your medication during the pre-taper.

Pre-Taper Goals:

*   Improved sleep.

*   Vast reduction or elimination of anxiety, fatigue and insomnia.

Lessening or elimination of other drug-induced side effects.

Below are the supplements you will take:

Neuro Endure Mini – **Take 1 tablet 3 times a day 5 hours apart**.

JNK Capsules – **Take 1 capsule in the mid-morning**.

Body Calm Daytime Relief

Body Calm Supreme With Melatonin or select

Body Calm Supreme Melatonin Free

DAY ONE THROUGH DAY THREE:

Use your Daily Journal and rate your anxiety, panic attacks, insomnia and any additional symptoms you may be experiencing. Rate them from 1 to 10, with number 10 being the worst and number 1 being no side effect or symptom remaining.

Rate your previous night's sleep first thing the next morning and your daytime anxiety just before bedtime of that day.

MORNING SUPPLEMENTS:

If you take your medication first thing in the morning, take the medication as usual, and 1 hour later take 1 Neuro Endure Mini. If you do not take the medication first thing in the morning, take the Neuro Endure Mini first thing. Never take supplements within 1 hour of medication.

JNK – Take 1 capsule in the mid-morning.

Body Calm Daytime Relief – 2 hours after the morning Neuro Endure Mini, take 1 capsule of Body Calm Daytime Relief. For the rest of the day and evening take 1 capsule every 2 to 4 hours.

If you found the morning JNK Capsule reduced your daytime

anxiety but the anxiety crept back in near noon, you can take an additional JNK Capsule anytime you wish.

You can take another JNK Capsule in the early evening if it is needed.

Bedtime

Body Calm Supreme– If you take medication at bedtime, take one capsule of the Body Calm Supreme one hour before taking your medication.

If you do not take medication at bedtime, take 1 capsule of Body Calm Supreme 15-minutes before going to bed. Take the supplements exactly as described here for 3 full days. If your anxiety levels are going down and your sleep is improving, remain with this schedule for at least 4 additional days.

How to Adjust the Supplements If Needed

JNK – Add additional capsules of the JNK supplement around noon. This usually handles any lingering side effect that might be related to anxiety, insomnia, etc. A few people take 9 capsules of the JNK each day; (3) morning, (3) noon and again (3) at around 4 pm, but that is rarely needed. If you do need to increase the JNK Capsules to more than once a day, try that for three days and then reduce back down to 3 capsules in the morning. Sometimes you only need the extra JNK Capsules for a day or two and you can then reduce back to the morning only and still feel well.

Body Calm Daytime Relief – You can take every 2 hours if needed. You can also increase the amount you take during the day to 2 capsules for each serving.

Body Calm Supreme – If you find you are sleeping much better when you go to sleep but you are still having difficulty going to sleep, take the Body Calm Supreme 1 hour earlier than you were taking it and add a second Body Calm Supreme 15-minutes before going to bed.

The concept of adjusting the supplements during the program is straightforward:

- If you felt an improvement after starting the JNK, but symptoms came back later in the day, take an additional JNK capsule about 4 hours after the morning JNK.

- If you responded well to the Body Calm Daytime Relief but the Body Calm Supreme you selected is not working as desired, change to the other Body Calm Supreme product. For some of us melatonin is fantastic and for others melatonin does not work. **If the Body Calm Daytime Relief is keeping you entirely chilled throughout the day, you can use the Body Calm Daytime Relief supplement at bedtime for sleep.**

If you started getting tired during the daytime, and this is new for you, try taking less of the Body Calm Daytime Relief.

If the Body Calm Daytime Relief helps but doesn't fully handle your symptoms, try taking 2 capsules instead of 1 or try taking it every 2 hours instead of every 4 hours.

- If anxiety always comes back at around noon each day, and it is not time to take the Body Calm Daytime Relief for another hour, adjust your schedule so you take 1 capsule of the Body Calm Daytime Relief at 11am.

- If anxiety or insomnia persists, try taking the extra JNK Capsule at noon and again around 4pm.

Make sure to keep your Daily Journal and graphs updated each day. The pre-taper is really that simple.

After 7 full days of the pre-taper, you are now ready to begin reducing the medication.

The key is to keep good notes or, at the very least, make a mental note of how you felt. You can adjust the supplements around as you like, but be consistent with how you adjust them.

If you feel a massive reduction of symptoms after taking the Neuro Endure Mini, you can adjust around the time you take it. Try and keep the time at least 4 hours apart though. You can try taking 2 tablets of the Neuro Endure Mini 3 times a day 5 hours apart. If the 2 tablets work well for you, you can change to the Neuro Endure and just break that tablet in half to consume the same amount that is found in the Neuro Endure Mini.

Chapter 10

Time Release Antidepressant Pre-Taper

Please Note: This pre-taper is for individuals taking a time-release antidepressant. Your brand may be called; extended release sustained release or any other name that means the antidepressant will metabolize slowly, over an extended period of time.

Starting Your Pre-Taper

If you have not read the entire chapter "General Pre-Tapering and Tapering Instructions," please do so before continuing with this chapter. Reading and understanding the chapter "General Pre-Tapering and Tapering Instructions" is vital before starting the pre-taper.

You may already be in withdrawal before you found The Road Back Program. Please hang in there; relief can come very quickly for you. Most people are never able to get off an antidepressant due to the head symptoms that are common with reducing this type of medication and the larger percentage of reduction that must be done because of the availability of dosages. It is too common to have reductions of 25% or more because the drugs only come in those dosages.

Your pre-taper is a little different than for an immediate release antidepressant.

The American Medical Association now acknowledges at least 10% of the people that try to get off an antidepressant will not be successful due to the withdrawal side effects. The 10% is probably higher with a time-release antidepressant. We want you to know this so you know it is not just you. Sorry to say, most physicians have never read the AMA report on antidepressant withdrawal and they have not realized that 1 out of every 10 of their patients they have prescribed an antidepressant to will have this withdrawal problem unless they begin doing something differently.

Head side effects are the ones that stop most people from being able to get off an antidepressant. An electrical brain zap, dizziness and other head symptoms are the problem. For The Road Back, these debilitating head side effects are easy to stop and stop quickly. If you have not started to taper the antidepressant yet, using this Antidepressant Pre-taper should stop the head symptoms from even starting. If you have already started to taper the antidepressant and have these head symptoms, the right type of omega 3 fish oil will get you back on your feet quickly.

The supplements required for the time release antidepressant program are the JNK Capsules, Omega 3 Supreme TG, Neuro Endure Mini and vitamin E.

At first look, you or your physician might ask, "what does vitamin E have to do with withdrawal" or "are you trying to tell me vitamin E will help with withdrawal side effects?"

Here is the answer – Vitamin E will not help with withdrawal symptoms at all. When a person takes omega 3 fish oil, the omega 3 will deplete vitamin E from the body and use the vitamin E to help for absorption. You will become deficient in vitamin E if you take fish oil daily and do not supplement with vitamin E. That is the only reason why vitamin E is in this program.

Make sure to keep your Daily Journal up-to-date and use graphs so you can visually see the changes taking place with you.

What to do:

1. Get with your prescribing physician and/or pharmacist and layout your drug taper schedule.

2. Plan out the second and third reduction of the medication as well at this point to ensure you are ready with the correct dosages of the drug.

Once you have read all of the pre-taper section proceed to the chapter, How to Taper Antidepressants and fully read it as well.

The Pre-Taper

For the next 7-days you will be doing your pre-taper. You do not reduce your antidepressant during the pre-taper, but, to state again, this is the time to also plan out the reduction phase of the drug which starts after the seven days of the pre-taper are completed.

Goal of Antidepressant Pre-taper

• If anxiety is present, have it eliminated

• If fatigue is present, have it eliminated

• If flu like symptoms are present, have them eliminated

• If depression is present, have it eliminated

• Eliminate all other antidepressant side effects

• Set up the body correctly to eliminate potential withdrawal symptoms.

The goal of the pre-taper may seem unobtainable to you at this moment, but after you experience a day to two of taking the supplements used with this program, you should begin to experience the changes we suggest will happen. It is not out of character for people to feel as though they are no longer even on an antidepressant as all side effects vanish quickly.

Supplements You Will Take:

JNK Capsules

Neuro Endure Mini

Omega 3 Supreme TG

Vitamin E

Anxiety or Insomnia

If you have daytime anxieties include the Body Calm Daytime Relief and if you have insomnia include one of the Body Calm Supreme supplements.

Fatigue

If you have fatigue, the Neuro Endure Mini should handle that rather well.

DAY ONE Action:

Rate your daytime anxiety, panic attacks, insomnia and other side effects. Use the Daily Journal and rate anxiety, sleep and any additional symptoms you may be experiencing from 1 to 10. Rate with number 10 being the worst and number 1 being no side effect or symptom remaining.

Rate the previous night's sleep first thing the next morning. Rate the daytime anxiety just before bedtime of that day.

If you take the antidepressant first thing in the morning, take the medication as normal and 1 hour later take the morning supplements.

How to do the Pre-Taper

Supplements:

JNK – Take 1 capsule of the JNK supplement in the mid-morning. You can take with or without food.

Omega 3 Supreme TG – Take 2 Omega 3 Supreme TG in the morning and 2 more at noon.

Vitamin E – Take 1 vitamin E along with the Omega 3 Supreme TG in the morning.

Neuro Endure Mini – Take 1 tablet 3 times a day 5 hours apart. Take first one in the morning.

Optional Supplements For Specific Conditions

Anxiety or Insomnia

Anxiety:

Body Calm Daytime Relief - 2 hours after the morning Neuro Endure

Mini, take 1 capsule of Body Calm Daytime Relief.

Take an additional capsule of Body Calm Daytime Relief every 2 to 4 hours during the day and evening.

You can increase the Body Calm Daytime Relief to 2 capsules if necessary.

You can also take the Body Calm Daytime Relief every 2 hours if necessary.

Body Calm Supreme With Melatonin or Melatonin Free – 15-minutes before bedtime take 1 capsule. If sleep has not improved within 3 days increase to 2 capsules.

Fatigue

If you have fatigue, the Neuro Endure Mini should handle it fine.

How to Adjust the Supplements if Needed

JNK – You can take 3 additional capsules in the afternoon if desired. The best way to judge if the second amount is needed would be; if the morning JNK makes a wonderful change in how you feel but around noon or so you feel a letdown.

Some people take 1 or 2 capsules at noon and that gets them over this period, while very few need 3 more capsules in the late day.

Neuro Endure Mini – You can take up to 4 tablets of the Neuro Endure Mini at a time. Only start with 1 tablet and only increase by 1 tablet every 7 days. When you reach the amount needed, you will know it by how you feel.

Neuro Endure Mini is formulated to be taken 3 times a day, starting in the morning and twice more during the day 5 hours apart. So, 1 tablet in the morning, 5 hours later another tablet and another tablet again in 5 hours.

The Neuro Endure Mini should make a massive positive change for you when you are taking the right amount for your body. Adjust it around if needed but try and take at least 4 hours apart.

Omega 3 Supreme TG – All head symptoms, except headaches, when coming off an antidepressant are handled by the Omega 3 Supreme TG. If you are feeling any symptoms in the head, increase the Omega 3 Supreme TG to 2 softgels in the morning and 2 additional softgels at noon. If symptoms persist after this increase, raise the amount of Omega 3 Supreme TG to 5 softgels in the morning and 5 at noon. A few people have needed to increase to 6 softgels in the morning and at noon to get the head symptoms under control. Once the head symptoms are back under control reduce the Omega 3 Supreme TG back down to the 3 softgels in the morning and the 3 softgels at noon. Check with your doctor before increasing the Omega 3 fish oil if you are taking heart medication or blood pressure medication.

Body Calm Daytime Relief – You can take as many as 2 capsules every 2-hours if needed.

Body Calm Supreme - Usually 1 capsule will do the trick for sleep. You can increase to 2 capsules. The capsule dissolves in 15-minutes after swallowing. If you need to take this supplement a little earlier that is fine. Remember, you can take 2 capsules if needed.

95

Finishing the Pre-Taper

Do the pre-taper for 7-full days. Do not cut the pre-taper short no matter how well you may feel after a few days. Give your body a chance to balance, give yourself the chance to fully experience relief before you tackle the reduction of the antidepressant.

If you wish to stay on the pre-taper for an extended time, that is fine to do, many have. You may have experienced extreme trauma the last time you tried to get off the antidepressant and the apprehension you may feel now is normal, not a mental disorder. This is your time; do not let yourself get rushed by your physician or by the information in this book. The drug manufacturer, the F.D.A., and even the American Medical Association state a gradual reduction of the medication is required. We cannot stress enough, take your time. This is when the tortoise beats the hare to the finish line.

If you have questions or need some help adjusting the supplements around send us an e-mail with your questions. INFO@THEROADBACK.ORG

Chapter 11

Immediate Release
Antidepressant Pre-Taper

Please Note: This pre-taper is for individuals taking an **Immediate Release** antidepressant.

Starting Your Pre-Taper

If you have not read the entire chapter "General Pre-Tapering and Tapering Instructions," please do so before continuing with this chapter. Reading and understanding the chapter "General Pre-Tapering and Tapering Instructions" is vital before starting the pre-taper.

You may already be in withdrawal before you found The Road Back Program. Please hang in there; relief can come very quickly for you. Most people are never able to get off an antidepressant due to the head symptoms that are common with reducing this type of medication.

Your pre-taper is a little different than for a time release antidepressant.

The American Medical Association now acknowledges at least 10% of the people that try to get off an antidepressant will not be successful due to the withdrawal side effects. The 10% is probably higher with a time-release antidepressant. We want you to know this so you know it is not just you. Sorry to say, most physicians have never read the AMA report on antidepressant withdrawal and they have not realized that 1 out of every 10 of their patients they have prescribed an antidepressant to will have this withdrawal problem unless they begin doing something differently.

Head side effects are the ones that stop most people from being able to get off an antidepressant. An electrical brain zap, dizziness and other head symptoms are the problem. For The Road Back, these debilitating head side effects are easy to stop and stop quickly. If you have not started to taper the antidepressant yet, using this Antidepressant Pre-taper should stop the head symptoms from even starting. If you have already started to taper the antidepressant and have these head symptoms, the right type of omega 3 fish oil will get you back on your feet quickly.

The supplements that are required for the immediate release antidepressant withdrawal program are the Neuro Endue Mini, JNK Capsules, Omega 3 Supreme TG, and vitamin E.

You or your physician might ask, "what does vitamin E have to do with withdrawal" or "are you trying to tell me vitamin E will help with withdrawal side effects?"

Here is the answer – Vitamin E will not help with withdrawal symptoms at all. When a person takes omega 3 fish oil, the omega 3 will deplete vitamin E from the body and use the vitamin E to help with absorption. You will become deficient in vitamin E if you take fish oil daily and do not supplement with vitamin E. That is the only reason why vitamin E is in this program.

Make sure to keep your Daily Journal up-to-date and use graphs so you can visually see the changes taking place with you.

What to do:

1. Get with your prescribing physician and/or pharmacist and layout your drug taper schedule.

2. Plan out the second and third reduction of the medication as well at this point to ensure you are ready with the correct dosages of the drug.

Once you have read all of the pre-taper section proceed to the chapter, How to Taper Antidepressants and fully read it as well.

The Pre-Taper

For the next 7-days you will be doing your pre-taper. You do not reduce your antidepressant during the pre-taper but, to state again, this is the time to also plan out the reduction phase of the drug which starts after the seven days of the pre-taper are completed.

Goal of Antidepressant Pre-taper

• If anxiety is present, have it eliminated

• If fatigue is present, have it eliminated

• If flu like symptom are present, have them eliminated

• If depression is present, have it eliminated

• Eliminate all other antidepressant side effects

• Set up the body correctly to eliminate potential withdrawal symptoms.

The goal of the pre-taper may seem unobtainable to you at this moment, but after you experience a day to two of taking the supplements used with this program, you should begin to experience the changes we suggest will happen. It is not out of character for people to feel as though they are no longer even on an antidepressant as all side effects vanish quickly.

Supplements You Will Take:

Neuro Endure Mini

JNK Capsules

Omega 3 Supreme TG

Vitamin E

Anxiety or Insomnia

If you have daytime anxieties include the Body Calm Daytime Relief and if you have insomnia include the Body Calm Supreme With Melatonin or use the Body Calm Supreme Melatonin Free.

Fatigue

If you have fatigue, you can increase the Neuro Endure Mini and it should handle that rather well.

DAY ONE Action:

Rate your daytime anxiety, panic attacks, insomnia and other side effects. Use the Daily Journal and rate anxiety, sleep and any additional symptoms you may be experiencing from 1 to 10. Rate with number 10 being the worst and number 1 being no side effect or symptom remaining.

Rate the previous night's sleep first thing the next morning. Rate the daytime anxiety just before bedtime of that day.

If you take the antidepressant first thing in the morning, take the medication as normal and 1 hour later take the morning supplements.

How to do the Pre-Taper

Supplements:

JNK – Take 1 capsule of the JNK supplement in mid-morning.

Omega 3 Supreme TG – Take 1 Omega 3 Supreme TG in the morning and 1 more at noon.

Vitamin E – Take 400 i.u. of vitamin E along with the Omega 3 Supreme TG in the morning.

Neuro Endure Mini – Take 1 tablet 3 times a day 5 hours apart.

Optional Supplements For Specific Conditions

Anxiety or Insomnia

Anxiety:

Body Calm Daytime Relief - 2 hours after the morning Neuro Endure Mini, take 1 capsule of Body Calm Daytime Relief.
Take an additional capsule of every 4 hours during the day and evening. You can increase to 2 capsules if necessary. You can also take the every 2 hours if necessary.

Body Calm Supreme With Melatonin or Melatonin Free – 15-minutes before bedtime take 1 capsule. If sleep has not improved within 3 days increase to 2 capsules.

Fatigue

If you have fatigue, the Neuro Endure Mini should handle it fine. You can increase to 4 tablets 3 times a day 5 hours apart if necessary.

How to Adjust the Supplements if Needed

JNK – You can take additional capsules in the afternoon if desired. The best way to judge if the second amount is needed would be; if the morning JNK makes a wonderful change in how you feel but around noon or so you feel a letdown.

Some people take 1 or 2 capsules at noon and that gets them over this period, although very few need more capsules in the late day.

Neuro Endure Mini – If you feel the need to increase, only increase by 1 tablet every 7 days. Once you feel a positive change to the Neuro Endure Mini do not increase any further.

Neuro Endure Mini is formulated to be taken 3 times a day, starting in the morning and twice more during the day, 5 hours apart. So, 1 tablet in the morning, 5 hours later another tablet and another tablet again in 5 hours.

Omega 3 Supreme TG – All head symptoms, except headaches, when coming off an antidepressant are handled by the Omega 3 Supreme TG. If you are feeling any symptoms in the head, increase the Omega 3 Supreme TG to 2 softgels in the morning and 2 additional softgels at noon. If symptoms persist after this increase, raise the amount of Omega 3 Supreme TG to 5 softgels in the morning and 5 at noon. A few people have needed to increase to 6 softgels in the morning and at noon to get the head symptoms under control. Once the head symptoms are back under control reduce the Omega 3 Supreme TG back down to the 3 softgels in the morning and the 3 softgels at noon. Check with your doctor before increasing the Omega 3 fish oil if you are taking heart medication or blood pressure medication.

Body Calm Daytime Relief – You can take as many as 2 capsules every 2-hours if needed.

Body Calm Supreme - Usually 1 capsule will do the trick for sleep. You can increase to 2 capsules. The capsule dissolves in 15-minutes after swallowing. If you need to take this supplement a little earlier that is fine.

Finishing the Pre-Taper

Do the pre-taper for 7-full days. Do not cut the pre-taper short no matter how well you may feel after a few days. Give your body a chance to balance, give yourself the chance to fully experience relief before you tackle the reduction of the antidepressant.

If you wish to stay on the pre-taper for an extended time, that is fine to do, many have. You may have experienced extreme trauma the last time you tried to get off the antidepressant and the apprehension you may feel now is normal, not a mental disorder.

This is your time; do not let yourself get rushed by your physician or by the information in this book. The drug manufacturer, the F.D.A., and even the American Medical Association state a gradual reduction of the medication is required. We cannot stress enough, take your time. This is when the tortoise beats the hare to the finish line.

If you need any assistance along the way or have any questions send an e-mail to info@theroadback.org

Chapter 12

Antipsychotic
Medication Pre-Taper

THE PRE-TAPER FOR an antipsychotic medication has changed more than any other medication type with recent scientific breakthroughs at The Road Back. The amount of nutritional supplements required has continued to drop dramatically with these discoveries and the ease a person can now get off an antipsychotic has dramatically improved.

Antipsychotics disrupt additional balances within the body and the drug created conditions need to be addressed. In the past years, antipsychotics were only prescribed for schizophrenia, bipolar, psychosis and extreme mental disturbances, but that is no longer the case. This edition of the book includes the recent breakthroughs that dramatically reduce the side effects and major symptoms associated with antipsychotic medication as well as the normal mental symptoms people may be experiencing that might prompt a physician to prescribe this class of medication initially.

Starting Your Pre-Taper

Now is the time to take a deep breath and relax. You may have suffered greatly from the medication in the past and you may be suffering from what appears to be side effects that will never go away. There is hope and there is a solution. Your body will be going through some changes during the pre-taper and those changes are positive changes. Your life is about to change for the better.

If you need assistance from a parent or a trusted friend, give them this book and have them work with you and help you through the daily procedures.

Your physician should also be supportive as well.

What to do:

1. Consult with your prescribing physician and/or pharmacist and layout your drug taper schedule.

2. Plan out the second and third reduction of the medication as well at this point to ensure you are ready with the correct dosages of the drug.

3. Once you have read all of the pre-taper section proceed to the chapter, How to Taper Antipsychotic Medication and fully read it as well.

The Pre-Taper

For the next 7-days you will be doing your pre-taper. You do not reduce your medication during the pre-taper, but, to state again, this is the time to also plan out the reduction phase of the drug which starts after the seven days of the

106

pre-taper are completed.

Goal of Pre-Taper

• Drastic reduction of all major side effects.

• If hearing voices, those completely gone.

• Mood swings stabilized.

Supplements you will take:

JNK

Neuro Endure Mini

Omega 3 Supreme TG

Body Calm Daytime Relief

Body Calm Supreme, either with or without melatonin

DAY ONE

Supplements

JNK Capsules – Take 2 of the JNK Capsules in the mid-morning, 2 more at noon and 2 more capsules around 6pm.

Neuro Endure Mini – Start with 1 tablet in the morning. Take the next tablet 5 hours later and a 3rd tablet 5 hours after the second tablet.

After 7 days of taking 1 tablet, you can increase to 2 tablets 3 times a day **if a positive change has not happened yet**. Increase by 1 tablet every 7 days until a positive change occurs. No need to exceed more than 4 tablets 3 times a day, 5 hours apart.

Most of you will respond to only 1 tablet. When positive change occurs do not increase further.

Omega 3 Supreme TG – Take 1 softgel in the morning and another softgel at noon. There is enough vitamin e in the fish oil softgel when you are only taking two softgels a day. You will not need additional vitamin E.

Body Calm Daytime Relief – Take 1 capsule throughout the day and into the evening. This should help keep the edge off. If needed, you can take the Body calm Daytime Relief every 2 hours and as many as 2 capsules if desired. If the Body Calm Daytime Relief is working very well for you during the daytime and you feel completely chilled, you can try taking the Body Calm Daytime Relief for sleep as well.

Body Calm Supreme – Take 1 or 2 capsules 15-minutes before bedtime. You can use the melatonin free formula or with melatonin. The formula with melatonin is stronger.

Refer to the chapter, Nutritionals Used on the Program for additional information about the supplements.

Make sure to keep your daily Journal and Daily Graphs. The pre-taper is really this simple. Do the pre-taper for 7 full days and then proceed to tapering off the medication.

If you have any questions or need guidance send an e-mail to info@theroadback.org

Chapter 13

ADD, ADHD
Medication And
Stimulants Pre-Taper

Starting Your Pre Taper

If you are wondering how you will feel once you are off the medication or during the withdrawal portion of the program, you are not alone and that is a normal question. Most people begin to feel a major improvement once they start the pre-taper and the rest feel a positive change once the medication begins to be reduced.

I am assuming you were prescribed this class of medication for Attention Deficit Disorder or Attention Deficit Hyperactivity Disorder. The pre-taper and the supplements used in this program will not only help eliminate withdrawal, but will probably give your body some basic nutrients it was lacking before the diagnosis and are probably one of the root causes of the symptoms you experienced.

What to do Next:

1. Consult with your prescribing physician and/or pharmacist and layout your drug taper schedule.

3. Plan out the second and third reduction of the medication as

well at this point to ensure you are ready with the correct dosages of the drug.

Once you have read all of the pre-taper section proceed to the chapter, How to Taper ADD, ADHD Medication and Stimulants and fully read it as well.

The Pre-Taper

For the next 7-days you will be doing your pre-taper. You do not reduce your medication during the pre-taper..

Goal of Pre-Taper Drastic reduction or elimination of all major side effects.

Supplements You Will Take

JNK Capsules

Neuro Endure Mini

Optional Supplements

ADHD medication is different from other psychoactive medications during withdrawal. You might alternate from being anxious and having insomnia one week and then fatigued and dull for the next few weeks and then back again to anxious and not able to sleep.

The JNK supplement might handle both ends of the spectrum but it may not be able to completely eliminate the anxiety, insomnia, fatigue and a dull feeling.

We recommend you have on hand the Body Calm Daytime Relief if you are prone to have anxiety in the daytime and Body Calm Supreme, with or without melatonin if insomnia is an issue for you currently.

Body Calm Daytime Relief

Body Calm Supreme With Melatonin

Or

Body Calm Supreme Melatonin Free

JNK Capsules – Take 1 capsule of the JNK in the mid-morning. Take with or without food.

Neuro Endure Mini – Take 1 tablet in the morning. Take a total of 3 tablets a day 5 hours apart.

Optional Supplements

Body Calm Daytime Relief – Taking 1 capsule every 4 hours will usually help keep you chilled out during the daytime. You can increase to 2 capsules if desired or take every 2 hours if needed.

Body Calm Supreme (With Melatonin or Melatonin Free) – Start with the 1 capsule 15-minutes before bedtime and give this amount 3 days. If your sleep is not what you desire increase to as much as 2 capsules. You might try taking 1 hour before bedtime as well.

Refer to the chapter, Nutritionals Used on The Road Back Program for additional information.

Make sure to keep your daily Journal and Daily Graphs. The pre-taper is really this simple. Do the pre-taper for 7 full days and then proceed to tapering off the medication.

If you have any questions or need assistance send us an e-mail to info@theroadback.org

Chapter 14

How To Taper Anti-Anxiety, Anticonvulsants, Benzodiazepine, And Sleep Medication

THE FDA HAS published approved guidelines for tapering off these medications. Those guidelines are what the authors published a decade ago and this approach is as effective now as it was in 1999.

Reduce the medication gradually and if side effects begin that are too severe, go back to the last dosage you were doing fine with, get stable again and then reduce the medication again, but this time at a slower reduction amount.

Gradual – Most of us take the word gradual to mean slowly, but there is a need to give a good example of gradual. Imaging you are in an airplane that is about to descend for the landing. What would you like that landing to be like? Would you prefer to not feel the decent and when the plane touches the runway you do not even feel the tires touch ground? This is a landing where I have heard the passengers cheer and thank the pilot when they get off the plane. This is also the gradual landing we want for you when reducing your medication.

"Gradual" when tapering off a medication would be; a slow and steady decent that does not jar and bump the person reducing the drug. Gradual would also be a speed of reduction that would allow the person to still function in life and reduce to a minimum the chance of withdrawal side effects.

If you agree with the above, this removes the idea of skipping days of the medication in order to reduce the dosage and get off the drug. Skipping days or alternating from a higher dosage to a lower dosage every other day is not gradual. One only needs to examine the half-life of the medication to establish that fact. You go into withdrawal every other day and feel an overdose effect the days you are going back up on the dosage.

Never Skip Days of the Drug

All drugs in this class come in completely different dosages and with some being in a time-release, the variances are too vast to list in a book of this type. We will first discuss what to do with a non-time release medication.

ONLY REDUCE MEDICATION EVERY 14-DAYS
Non-Time Release Medication

If you are taking a non-time release medication, reduce the medication as close to 5% as possible. I understand the 5% is an arbitrary number but this is what most have found to work well.

With most medications being different there is no way for us to describe each one and your physician and pharmacist should be involved in this process regardless.

Some medications can be compounded into exact and precise

reductions. Compounding is when the pharmacist takes the medication and grinds it to a powdered form and then encapsulates to a new dosage. This is the ideal way to reduce all medications but some cannot be compounded and the cost can also be out of reach for some individuals.

With your pharmacist, see if purchasing a pill slicer will work for you. These typically cost about $5 at a pharmacy.

You can also purchase a relative low cost digital scale that will measure milligram amounts.

Talk with your pharmacist about putting the medication in a solution for measuring reductions. Some medications dissolve well and can be crushed and put in water and then you pour out of a flask the reduction amount.

An experienced pharmacist will be of great value to you during this process.

Time Release or Extended Release Medication

When it comes to reducing medication that is time release, the process needs to be a little different with the program. Sometimes time release medications are also offered in a non-time release form and it is best to cross-over to the non-time release form of the drug. Your physician and pharmacist are the ones to guide you through how to take the medication. Cross over to the non-time release form of the medication if that is at all possible. The cross- over would be the first reduction.

How to Adjust Supplements During the Taper

Keeping good notes with your Daily Journal during the pre-taper is worth its weight in gold during the tapering of the medication.

A rule of thumb: The supplement that got rid of a side effect or symptom during the pre-taper is the supplement to increase during the taper if that symptom returns while tapering off the drug. An example of this can be made with the JNK Capsules.

If all of your anxiety vanished during the pre-taper after starting the Neuro Endure Mini and anxiety creeps back when you start reducing the medication, increase the Neuro Endure Mini by 1 tablet for each serving. When the anxiety vanishes again, reduce the Neuro Endure Mini back to 1 tablet per serving.

You can increase any of the supplements to eliminate the side effects again. After the side effect diminishes reduce the supplement back down again to the amount you were taking.

If you experience withdrawal side effects every time you reduce the medication increase the supplements the day before you reduce the drug, wait 4 days to ensure there is no withdrawal and then reduce the supplements back down again.

If you are reducing a time-release medication you should ALWAYS increase the supplements the day before you reduce the drug. Your reduction amount will be higher than desirable and increasing the supplements will be required to help eliminate the withdrawal.

116

If the information above is not making a smooth and relative withdrawal free program for you, it is time to reduce the drug at a slower pace.

We do not advise switching from one drug to another drug because the new one has a longer half-life. This does not work and will cause more problems and symptoms than you currently are experiencing. Some people promote crossing over to Valium because of the longer half-life. DO NOT DO THIS.

Reread and keep in mind the chapter, Nutritionals Used in The Road Back Program for tips and how to increase the supplements.

Reducing the medication is actually the easy part of the program.

Note: If you have had difficulty reducing the medication in the past, compounding the drug for a 2% reduction is advised. Reduce every 14-days, have success and then try reducing by 5% every 14-days.

If this is your first attempt tapering the medication, start with a 5% reduction, reduce again in 14-days and repeat at the 5% reduction two additional times. If successful, you can try a further increase of reduction, but that is not advised. If withdrawal side effects begin, go back to the last dosage you were doing fine with and for the next reduction, reduce at a more gradual rate.

Chapter 15

How To Taper
Antidepressants

THE FDA HAS published approved guidelines for tapering off these medications. Those guidelines are what the authors published a decade ago and this approach is as effective now as it was in 1999. The American Medical Association published a report in 2010 acknowledging at least 10% of the population will not be able to get off their antidepressant because of the withdrawal side effects. One particular side effect associated with antidepressant withdrawal is the "brain zaps." This is an electrical jolt that runs from the base of the neck to the base of the skull and the jolt can happen several times a day or non-stop.

The Road Back program is the pioneer in this area and we were the ones that found the solution years ago. Omega 3 fish oil is the key to get rid of the brain zaps as well as to never allow them to start. Using the correct omega 3 fish oil is critical and you need to know just any fish oil will not do the trick. It takes an omega 3 fish oil made from sardines and the EPA to DHA ratio content needs to be specific. Flax seed will not work; please do not waste your time and the unneeded trauma. If you are a vegetarian it is time to take a break if you want to have a chance of eliminating the brain zaps. To be blunt, it is time to decide which is worse for you; an antidepressant or fish oil for a short time.

We only recommend Omega 3 Supreme TG, a fish oil that is distilled and brought back to the true natural form of the oil of fish.

Reducing the Medication

Reduce the medication gradually and if side effects begin that are too severe, go back to the last dosage you were doing fine with, get stable again and then reduce the medication again, but this time at a slower reduction amount.

The above can seem too basic and too easy to understand for it to be misinterpreted. However, that is not the case.

Gradual – Most of us take the word gradual to mean slowly, but there is a need to give a good example of gradual. Imaging you are in an airplane that is about to descend for the landing. What would you like that landing to be like? Would you prefer to not feel the decent and when the plane touches the runway you do not even feel the tires touch ground. This is a landing where I have heard the passengers cheer and thank the pilot when they get off the plane. This is also the gradual landing we want for you when reducing your medication.

Gradual when tapering off a medication would be; a slow

and steady decent that does not jar and bump the person reducing the drug. Gradual would also be a speed of reduction that would allow the person to still function in life and reduce to a minimum the chance of withdrawal side effects.

If you agree with the above, this removes the idea of skipping days of the medication in order to reduce the dosage and get off the drug. Skipping days or alternating from a higher dosage to a lower dosage every other day is not gradual. One only needs to examine the half-life of the medication to establish that datum. You go in withdrawal every other day and feel an overdose effect the days you are going back up on the dosage.

Reduce the antidepressant as close to 10% with each reduction as possible. With this approach 10 reductions and you are off the antidepressant.

Never Skip Days of the Drug

All drugs in this class come in completely different dosages and with some being in a time-release the variances are too vast to list in a book of this type.

We will first take what to do with a non-time release medication.

ONLY REDUCE MEDICATION EVERY 14-DAYS

Non-Time Release Medication

If you are taking a non-time release medication, reduce the medication at the smallest reduction possible. We understand the "smallest reduction possible" is an arbitrary and we assure you it will be interpreted differently by many physicians and pharmacists.

With most medications being different there is no way for us to describe each one and your physician and pharmacist should be involved in this process regardless.

Some medications can be compounded in to exact and precise reductions. Compounding is when the pharmacist takes the medication and grinds it to a powdered form and then encapsulates to a new dosage. This is the ideal way to reduce all medications but some cannot be compounded and the cost can also be out of reach for some individuals.

With your pharmacist, see if purchasing a pill slicer will work for you. You can also purchase a relative low cost digital scale that will measure milligram amounts. Talk with your pharmacist about putting the medication in a solution for measuring reductions. Some medications dissolve well and can be crushed and put in water and then you pour out of a flask the reduction amount.

An experienced pharmacist will be of great value to you during this process.

Remember, as close to 10% reduction as you can do.

Time Release or Extended Release Medication

When it comes to reducing medication that is time release, the process needs to be a little different with the program. Sometimes time release medications are also offered in a non-time release form and it is best to cross-over to the non-time release form of the drug. Your physician and pharmacist are the ones to guide you through how to take the medication. Cross over to the non- time release form of the medication if that is at all possible. Count the cross-over as the first reduction and do not lower the medication for 14-days.

You have specific dosages of a time release antidepressant. **DO NOT OPEN THE CAPSUES AND COUNT THE BALLS.** Over the years, many people sent us an e-mail about how well they were doing with removing the balls from the capsule. Invariably, each of them contacted us again but this time in full withdrawal and it took an extended period of time to get them back on track again. Please, do not taper an antidepressant in this manner.

DO NOT OPEN THE CAPSUE AND POUR THE BALLS IN LIQUID AND REDUCE GRADUALLY BY REMOVING A PORTION OF THE LIQUID EACH DAY. This will cause an overdose. A time release is designed to slowly enter the body, not all at once.

Follow the pre-taper precisely for Time Release Antidepressants. Go to the next available dosage of the antidepressant when you have felt stable for at least 5 days and 14-days have passed since the last reduction.

How to Adjust Supplements During the Taper

Keeping good notes with your daily Journal during the pre-taper is worth its weight in gold during the tapering of the medication.

A rule of thumb: The supplement that got rid of a side effect or symptom during the pre-taper is the supplement to increase during the taper if that symptom returns while tapering off the drug. An example of this can be made with the Neuro Endure Mini.

If all of your anxiety vanished during the pre-taper after starting the Neuro Endure Mini and anxiety creeps back when you start reducing the medication, increase the Neuro Endure Mini to 2 tablets per serving. When the anxiety vanishes again, reduce the Neuro Endure Mini back to 1 tablet per serving.

You can increase any of the supplements to eliminate the side effects again. After the side effect diminishes, reduce the supplement back down again to the amount you were taking.

If you experience withdrawal side effects every time you reduce the medication increase the supplements the day before you reduce the drug, wait 4 days to ensure there is no withdrawal and then reduce the supplements back down again.

If the information above is not making a smooth and relative withdrawal free program for you, it is time to reduce the drug at a slower pace.

Reread and keep in mind the chapter, Nutritionals Used in The Road Back Program for tips and how to increase the supplements.

Reducing the medication is actually the easy part of the program now.

If you have any problems or questions, send an e-mail to info@theroadback.org

Chapter 16

How To Taper Antipsychotic Medication

THE FDA HAS published approved guidelines for tapering off these medications. Those guidelines are what the authors published a decade ago and this approach is as effective now as it was in 1999.

If you are taking Cogentin along with an antipsychotic drug, you need to rotate the drug being reduced. Start by reducing the antipsychotic, wait 14-days and then reduce the Cogentin, wait 14-days and then reduce the antipsychotic drug again, and repeat this approach back and forth until off both medications.

Reducing the Medication

Reduce the medication gradually and if side effects begin that are too severe, go back to the last dosage you were doing fine with, get stable again and then reduce the medication again, but this time at a slower reduction amount. The above can seem too basic and too easy to understand for it to be misinterpreted. However, that is not the case.

Gradual – Most of us take the word gradual to me slowly, but there is a need to give a good example of gradual. Imaging you are in an airplane that is about to descend for the landing. What would you like that landing to be like? Would you prefer to not feel the decent and when the plane touches the runway you do not even feel the tires touch ground. This is a landing where I have heard the passengers cheer and thank the pilot when they get off the plane. This is also the gradual landing we want for you when reducing your medication.

Gradual when tapering off a medication would be; a slow and steady decent that does not jar and bump the person reducing the drug. Gradual would also be a speed of reduction that would allow the person to still function in life and reduce to a minimum the chance of withdrawal side effects.

If you agree with the above, this removes the idea of skipping days of the medication in order to reduce the dosage and get off the drug. Skipping days or alternating from a higher dosage to a lower dosage every other day is not gradual. One only needs to examine the half-life of the medication to establish that datum. You go in withdrawal every other day and feel an overdose effect the days you are going back up on the dosage.

Never Skip Days of the Drug

All drugs in this class come in completely different dosages and with some being in a time-release the variances are too vast to list in a book of this type.

We will first take what to do with a non-time release medication.

ONLY REDUCE MEDICATION EVERY 14-DAYS Non-Time Release Medication

If you are taking a non-time release medication, reduce the medication at the smallest reduction possible. We understand the "smallest reduction possible" is an arbitrary and we assure you it will be interpreted differently by many physicians and pharmacists.

With most medications being different there is no way for us to describe each one and your physician and pharmacist should be involved in this process regardless. Some medications can be compounded into exact and precise reductions. Compounding is when the pharmacist takes the medication and grinds it to a powdered form and then encapsulates to a new dosage. This is the ideal way to reduce all medications but some cannot be compounded and the cost can also be out of reach for some individuals.

With your pharmacist, see if purchasing a pill slicer will work for you. You can also purchase a relatively low cost digital scale that will measure milligram amounts.

Talk with your pharmacist about putting the medication in a solution for measuring reductions. Some medications dissolve well and can be crushed and put in water and then you pour out of a flask the reduction amount.

An experienced pharmacist will be of great value to you during this process.

Time Release or Extended Release Medication

When it comes to reducing medication that is time release, the process needs to be a little different with the program. Sometimes time release medications are also offered in a non-time release form and it is best to cross-over to the non-time release form of the drug. Your physician and pharmacist are the ones to guide you through how to take the medication. Cross over to the non-time release form of the medication if that is at all possible. Count the cross-over as a reduction and do not reduce the medication for 14-days.

DO NOT OPEN THE CAPSULE AND REMOVE THE BALLS.

How to Adjust Supplements During the Taper

If you experience withdrawal side effects every time you reduce the medication, increase the supplements the day before you reduce the drug, wait 4 days to ensure there is no withdrawal and then reduce the supplements back down again.

Reducing the medication is actually the easy part of the program now.

Note: If you have had difficulty reducing the medication in the past, compounding the drug for a 5% reduction is advised. Reduce every 14-days, have success and then try reducing by 5% every 14-days.

If this is your first attempt tapering the medication, start with a 10% reduction, reduce again in 14-days and repeat at the 10% reduction two additional times. If successful, you can try a further increase of reduction, but that is not advised. If withdrawal side effects begin, go back to the last dosage you were doing fine with and for the next reduction, reduce at a more gradual rate.

Chapter 17

How To Taper
ADD, ADHD And
Stimulant Medication

THE FDA HAS published approved guidelines for tapering off these medications. Those guidelines are what I published a decade ago and this approach is as effective now as it was in 1999.

Reducing this class of medication is rather straightforward and usually does not cause a problem.

Reducing the Medication

Reduce the medication gradually and if side effects begin that are too severe, go back to the last dosage you were doing fine with, get stable again and then reduce the medication again, but this time at a slower reduction amount.

The above can seem too basic and too easy to understand for it to be misinterpreted. However, that is not the case.

Gradual – Most of us take the word gradual to me slowly, but there is a need to give a good example of gradual. Imaging you are in an airplane that is about to descend for the landing. What would you like that landing to be like? Would you prefer to not feel the decent and when the plane touches the runway you do not even feel the tires touch ground? This is a landing where I have heard the passengers cheer and thank the pilot when they get off the plane. This is also the gradual landing we want for you when reducing your medication.

Gradual when tapering off a medication would be; a slow and steady decent that does not jar and bump the person reducing the drug. Gradual would also be a speed of reduction that would allow the person to still function in life and reduce to a minimum the chance of withdrawal side effects.

If you agree with the above, this removes the idea of skipping days of the medication in order to reduce the dosage and get off the drug. Skipping days or alternating from a higher dosage to a lower dosage every other day is not gradual. One only needs to examine the half-life of the medication to establish that datum. You go in withdrawal every other day and feel an overdose effect the days you are going back up on the dosage.

Never Skip Days of the Drug

All drugs in this class come in completely different dosages and with most being in a time-release the variances are too vast to list in a book of this type. We will first take what to do with a non-time release medication.

ONLY REDUCE MEDICATION EVERY 14 DAYS

Non-Time Release Medication

If you are taking a non-time release medication, reduce the medication as near to 10% as possible. You can get a pill slicer from a pharmacy to help with this. Every 14-

days reduce the drug by another 10%. After 10 reductions of the drug you are drug free.

Time Release or Extended Release Medication

There are specific dosages the drug is available in as a time release. After 7 days of the pretaper, you reduce the drug to the next lower available dosage. Every 14-days you should be able to reduce the drug again to the next available lower dosage.

Continue with this method until completely off the drug.

DO NOT OPEN THE CAPSULE AND REMOVE THE BALLS.

How to Adjust Supplements During the Taper

Keeping good notes with your Daily Journal during the pre-taper is worth its weight in gold during the tapering of the medication.

A rule of thumb: You should not have a need to adjust the supplements at all during the taper. You may need to adjust the time you take the afternoon or evening supplement but only if a symptom happens to start just a little earlier than the normal time you take the supplement.

Quite often, this type of medication is used for energy, study problems and memory. Don't be surprised it you have more energy, a better concentration level and improved memory as the drug goes away and the supplements have a better chance to influence the body.

This class of a drug over activates the brain JNK gene and this over activation begins to kill off brain cells.

The Neuro Endure Mini should do you wonders.

Chapter 18

How To Taper
Off Multiple
Medications

What to Do If You Are Taking Multiple Drugs

With our breakthroughs this past year, people are now able to taper off more than one medication at a time. The reformulated JNK Capsules and Neuro Endure have made this possible and this new breakthrough cuts the time it takes a person to be medication free dramatically.

There are still some things that need to be watched when reducing more than one medication at a time.

The medications that can be reduced at the same time are: ADD, ADHD, stimulants, antidepressants and antipsychotics can be reduced at the same time. Any combination of these medications can be reduced simultaneously. **Alternate their reductions every 14-days.** An example of this would be:

• Reduce the antidepressant

• 7 days later reduce the antipsychotic

• 7 days later reduce the antidepressant again

• 7 days later reduce the antipsychotic again

This still gives 14-days before the dosage of a specific medication is reduced and if withdrawal side effects begin, it makes it easier to tell which drug reduction is causing the problem.

If you are also taking a benzodiazepine, anti-anxiety drug or sleep medication, taper these drugs first, before you reduce any other class of drug. The antidepressants, antipsychotics, ADD, ADHD, stimulants increase the clearance time of the benzodiazepines by as much as 50% and if you reduce these other drugs first you will go in withdrawal with the benzodiazepine, even though the benzodiazepine dosage was not reduced. You can read the chapter, The Science, for more information on this.

Pre-Taper for More Than One Drug

Read through the pre-taper chapters for each drug you want to taper off and use the required supplements and the instructions on how to take each supplement. You simply combine the programs.

Tapering off multiple medications is now as easy as tapering off one! Welcome to the New Road Back Program and we thank the people that paved the way for this advancement.

Chapter 19

What To Do

If You Are Already In
Withdrawal Or Quit Your Medication
Cold Turkey

In Withdrawal Already

The key to handling withdrawal side effects when you begin to reduce the medication is: **Put Control Back in the Process Again**.

Roughly 80% of the people who begin The Road Back Program have already started to taper off their medication or have gone off their medication abruptly and are experiencing withdrawal side effects. The recommendations or suggestions offered in this chapter come from years of experience assisting these individuals.

First, it is not YOU. That may be difficult to grasp at first, but in time, you will come to understand it was not you; it was the withdrawal side effect.

Immediately do the following if you have abruptly stopped your medication or are reducing the medication and you are having withdrawal side effects:

• Inform the prescribing physician

• Go to the pre-taper chapter in this book that covers your medication.

• Start the supplements in the pre-taper immediately

• If you are or were taking an antidepressant and you have head symptoms or an electrical jolt type of sensation, go to any store that sells vitamins and purchase a bottle of omega 3 fish oil. Look at the back label of the bottle and look for the highest amount of EPA content. This should get you some relief quickly, but make sure you get the Omega 3 Supreme TG from Neuro Genetic Solutions (www.shop.neurogeneticsolutions.com) for a complete solution. You will need to take around 1,500 mg of the EPA, so expect to take quite a few of the softgels from a local vitamin store. Most stores only sell omega 3 fish oil with low EPA amounts.

Relief should come shortly after you start the pre-taper supplements. I understand you may have already quit the medication and you are not actually doing a pre-taper now. Just start taking the supplements as described in the pre-taper and follow the directions as outlined in that chapter.

The supplements are formulated to work quickly, even when you have quit cold turkey.

Medication Decisions

You need to make a decision rather quickly about the medication. **I understand some of you absolutely refuse to go back on the medication or to go back up in dosage, but I still need to give you my viewpoint. This is only my viewpoint and should not be taken as**

138

medical advice.

If you have gone off the drug cold turkey and it has been more than one week since you stopped the drug, going back on the drug may not help. It may compound the situation. Not going back on the drug and doing a slow taper may be the only thing that will help. This is a flip of the coin and I do wish there was a better answer for you.

Start the pre-taper supplements and continue taking them for 45-days after you feel well again. Use the supplements based on the drug you were taking.

If it has been less than one week since you stopped the drug cold turkey, go back on the drug to the last dosage you were doing your best at, and do the pre-taper for that type of medication and gradually reduce the drug from that point.

You may feel this approach moves you backwards but it should get you off the drug and feeling well once again.

- If you are reducing the medication and you are experiencing withdrawal side effects, you need to determine the severity of the side effects. If the side effects are too strong, go back up to the last dosage when you were doing better. Start the pre-taper, get stable again and then gradually reduce the medication.

- If the side effects are on the mild side, quit reducing for now, start the pre-taper for the drug you are taking, after using the supplements for 7-days of the pre-taper, continue with the taper and supplements.

There is really no need to expand on this further. You may feel like death warmed over, but the options are few and they are basic. Keep in mind, how you feel is the drug and that it is not you. Make sure to inform your physician of any choice you make.

Chapter 20

Once Off All
Medication

CONGRATULATIONS! If anyone ever deserved a celebration party for an accomplishment, it is you. You not only made it off your medication, but also adhered to a schedule most other people have never had to confront. Only you can know what I mean.

As stated earlier in this book, you should continue taking all supplements for 45 days after the last dosage of the medication. It takes about 20 days for the liver enzymes used to metabolize the medication to return to a normal state, and depending on your own DNA, about 19 days for the medication to fully clear your body.

Continue writing in your Daily Journal during this ending of the program.

The supplements used during the program are not addictive and there is no withdrawal from these natural products. However, if you were lacking the nutrients found in a specific supplement and you discontinue using it, you may feel a letdown or a negative change. This would be the same feeling any person would have, even if they have never used these medications.

Omega 3 is needed in our diet. The human body needs an adequate amount of vitamins, minerals, and amino acids from a food source to work at an optimum level. If there were one supplement you would continue taking after the 45-days have passed, it would be Omega 3 Supreme TG fish oil.

Once off all medication for 45 days, it is advisable to get a complete physical exam with specific attention to hormones, adrenals, your immune system and insulin/glucose: an all-natural treatment, by a healthcare provider who fully understands that this intricate system is needed.

We strongly urge you to keep taking the JNK Capsules you have used during the program for the full 45-days after the last dosage of your medication. The JNK gene needs to be held in check for the body to have time to heal.

What to Do With Supplements

After you are off the medication for around 20 days, you may need to begin reducing some of the supplements.

Neuro Endure Mini – If you begin to feel to energized, you can reduce the Neuro Endure Mini to 1 tablet a day.

Body Calm Supplements – If you begin to feel tired during the daytime, it may be time to lower the amount of Body Calm Daytime Relief or Body Calm Supreme used at bedtime.

If you are going to lower either of these supplements, lower the Body Calm Daytime Relief first. Reduce slowly until the tiredness goes away. Keep your Daily Journal filled out each day. If the tiredness goes away by reducing or eliminating the daytime use of the Body Calm Daytime Relief, keep taking the Body Calm Supreme exactly as you have been.

Omega 3 Supreme TG – If you are taking 1 of the Omega 3 in the morning and at noon, you can reduce the Omega 3 down to 1 softgel in the morning.

If any head symptoms reappear, increase the Omega 3 back up.

Once again, congratulations on completing The Road Back Program and may your journey in life from this point forward be ever-expanding.

Chapter 21

What Can Be Done If You Have Never Taken Psychoactive Medication

If you are suffering from anxiety, stress that does not seem to end, fatigue or a host of symptoms, you absolutely have an alternative to psychoactive medication.

First: Get a complete physical and have the physician rule out all disease or illness.

There can be life events that were the direct cause of depression, anxiety, stress, fatigue and more. Usually, these feelings go away on their own in a matter of days or weeks without you doing anything other than letting some time pass.

If you lost your job and no matter how hard you search you can't find gain-full employment, which is depressing and stressful on all of us. It does not mean you now have an illness as some would like to make you believe. If you found the job you were looking for the depression and stress would vanish overnight. The answer is a job that pays what you need. You do not suddenly have a lifelong chemical imbalance due to unemployment.

145

These medications are strong, some are truly addicting, and all of the drugs are life altering. The question is how your life will be altered.

When depression, anxiety, stress, and/or fatigue begin, other factors also play a role in general health. Levels of hormones, adrenals, glucose, cortisol and other functions can become drained, imbalanced or overly stimulated. Psychoactive medications, in part, are designed to regulate all of these functions to some degree, but they ultimately affect these functions by altering other chemicals in the brain and body. Read the chapter, Drug Side Effects again if needed to gain a full understanding of the risk/reward.

Second: If you are diagnosed with a disease or illness, make sure the diagnosis is from an objective test – not a subjective analysis. As of this writing, all mental disorders are diagnosed with subjective tests.

Later in this chapter you will find possible solutions for symptoms you may be experiencing. One example is using the JNK Capsules, Body Calm Daytime Relief, and Body Calm Supreme for anxiety symptoms. These supplements do not cure disease or illness. With that in mind, if you feel the anxiety vanish once you begin using these supplements, you must not have had an Anxiety Disorder.

If you were diagnosed with chronic fatigue syndrome, take the JNK supplement and Neuro Endure Mini, and if you no longer feel the fatigue, you were misdiagnosed. Misdiagnoses can and does happen more often than not.

If a diagnosis of ADHD is presented, then you take JNK Capsules and Neuro Endure Mini. Again, these supplements do not cure or prevent disease or illness. If you feel the major positive changes after using these supplements, your body was just lacking those nutrients.

If you are hearing voices, experiencing ringing in the ears, seem to be manic and then feel depressed and you take the JNK Capsules and the Neuro Endure Mini, and those symptoms vanish, you were never bipolar, schizophrenic: you greatly lacked the nutrients found in those supplements.

Good-meaning, well-intentioned physicians often feel like they must prescribe psychoactive medication or face the threat of malpractice. One senior partner in a law firm refused to even read this book. Why? His answer was, "If there is a way to taper off psychiatric drugs, we would no longer have a case."

If you receive a clean bill of health from your physician, there are suggestions and probable solutions.

Read the chapter, Nutritionals Used on The Road Back Program and locate the supplement/s that pertains to how you feel. The supplements work quickly and you will probably experience relief faster than you ever imagined.

If you have just lost a loved one, there are no supplements or medications that will replace the loss. The most a psychoactive medication will do is deaden the feelings experienced because of the loss. The most a good supplement will do is assist the body to not succumb to the continued drain put on it because of the feeling of loss.

The Road Back of course, is unable to handle the life reason for anxiety, stress, depression or even fatigue. However, we can assist your body to not succumb to the physical stressors being put on it daily from emotional trauma.

Hundreds of clinical trials have shown that people with anxiety; stress, fatigue and depression have low levels of amino acids, vitamins, minerals, antioxidant levels and more. These clinical trials point to the fact that a person will suffer a depletion of these vital nutrients if they are put under enough stress or duress for a period of time.

Our goal here is to point out a few things you can do to help your body maintain general health and well-being while you address the real reason for the problem you are experiencing.

If an emotion continues beyond some arbitrary "they should be over it by now" time period, psychoactive medications come into play. Neither these drugs nor supplements will help you "realize" or have an "earth shattering realization" about why you have felt that way for such a long time or remove the loss you feel. They will not.

Psychoactive medication may block the emotion, but the emotion will need to be dealt with at some time in the future, unless you just wish to feel "flat- lined" forever. Most people tell us, in hindsight, they would have been better off dealing with the emotion when it happened, instead of putting it off for months or years and then dealing with the emotion on top of the drug withdrawal.

This is why The Road Back suggests using a few supplements. Again, the supplements are not going to solve the problem or underlying condition. They will only help maintain the body's general health and well-being and give you the chance to address the original problem.

Chapter 22

FREQUENTLY ASKED QUESTIONS

THIS CHAPTER MAINLY addresses questions about the supplements used on the program. Reducing the medication is fairly straightforward. You reduce the drug slowly and if side effects become too unbearable, go back to the last dosage you were doing fine with, get stable and the next time you reduce the drug, reduce it slower.

The Neuro Endure Mini will likely be the one supplement that brings the most change for you and the one supplement that gets rid of most withdrawal side effects.

Always start by only taking 1 Neuro Endure Mini 3 times a day 5 hours apart. From there you can adjust this supplement a little.

Let's say you are doing great most of the day but anxiety still comes back at 5pm and the next Neuro Endure Mini is not scheduled to take until 6pm. Take the Neuro Endure Mini at 4:30pm and see if that stops the 5pm anxiety from starting. The Neuro Endure Mini will tablet will completely dissolve within 30-minutes after you take the tablet and this may be all you need to do to fix the 5pm anxiety.

You can also increase the Neuro Endure Mini – You may do better taking 2 or 3 tablets, 3 times a day 5 hours apart.

You may do best taking 1 tablet in the morning and 2 tablets the second time you take the Neuro Endure Mini. It is ok to experiment with this. Keep good notes of how your major symptoms come and go during the daytime and adjust the Neuro Endure Mini accordingly.

When you experience a very positive change with the Neuro Endure Mini; that is the sign to not increase it further. Too much of a good thing is not what we are going for here.

JNK Capsules – The JNK capsules were introduced to the program mid-2010 and were a major breakthrough at that time for symptoms relief.

With the introduction of the Neuro Endure Mini the JNK capsules are not the predominate supplement any longer. It is still as effective as ever but with the Neuro Endure Mini addition, you no longer need to take as much of the JNK capsules.

Taking 1 JNK Capsule is all that is needed now instead of 3 capsules. Also changed, take the JNK Capsule in the mid-morning now. Take this supplement anywhere between your morning wake up and your normal lunchtime.

You can increase the JNK Capsules if you feel the need to do that. You can take as much as 3 capsules 3 times a day.

The best way to tell if more JNK is needed is by evaluating how you feel after taking the 1 JNK Capsule in the morning. If the morning JNK reduces any symptoms a little but not completely, try increasing by 1 capsule.

You can take additional JNK's in the afternoon and the evening as well. Decide if you should take more of the JNK based on symptoms, symptoms returning at specific times etc.

Most everyone will do perfectly fine with only one JNK each mid-morning so give this at least 7 days before you start adjusting the JNK around and start taking more.

Those of you tapering from an antidepressant or antipsychotic drug that have gained weight will likely be the candidates that will benefit from using additional JNK Capsules. Don't be surprised if you actually begin to lose some weight with this addition as well if you are overweight.

Body Calm Daytime Relief – If this supplement is what your body needs it will feel like true magic. A sign this is the right supplement for you will be; reduction of depression, reduction of anxiety, a more calm feeling and less agitation.

You can take 1 or 2 capsules at a time and you can take this supplement every 2 to 4 hours.

If the Body Calm Daytime Relief is that magical for you I suggest you try it as well at bedtime for sleep. Take 1 or 2 capsules 15-minutes before bedtime. If you awake in the middle of the night you can take additional capsules.

Adrenalpin – This supplement is often overlooked and overlooked by myself as well when assisting people. It was originally formulated to be used only when a person experienced anxiety first

Thing in the morning and the anxiety would fade away a little near noontime but then come back again at noon with full force. This is still the time to use the Adrenalpin but feedback from people has shown the Adrenalpin is quite effective for daytime anxiety even if it does not start, fade and return near noontime.

If the other supplements are not able to completely crack through the daytime anxiety, keep the Adrenalpin in mind. You would take 1 capsule in the mid-morning and 1 more in the mid-afternoon with a little food.

Omega 3 Supreme TG – I seriously doubt you will need to take more than 2 softgels in the morning and 2 at noon for the head symptoms when tapering an antidepressant but you can increase to as many as 4 softgels morning and noon if needed.

As soon as the head symptoms have left, reduce back down again.

When Reducing Medication

Sometimes when you reduce a medication side effects will still begin. If this is happening to you I suggest you increase the supplements the day before you lower the dosage of your drug.

You might increase the Neuro Endure Mini by 1 tablet, increase how much and often you take the JNK, and Body Calm Daytime Relief. If tapering an antidepressant and head symptoms always start, increase the Omega 3 Supreme TG the day before lowering the antidepressant.

Chapter 23

The Science

INTRODUCTION

The Road Back Program and the Development of the Program:

1. There are basic common denominators of psychotropic drug side effects.

2. How our individual DNA affects drug metabolism.

3. The effect of psychotropic medication within the Hypothalamic-Pituitary-Adrenal Axis and immune system.

4. Utilizing DNA clinical trials, test subject trials and psychotropic drug clinical trials to formulate specific nutritional products to eliminate, reduce or avert withdrawal side effects, while not creating drug/supplement interactions.

This research and development complexity has been transformed into an easy to understand, systematic program, which allows an individual to taper off their medication while alleviating a vast percentage of the debilitating side effects of withdrawal.

155

The sequence of this program and the application of each step is the key to success. Your patient will not begin to reduce a medication until the pre- taper is complete. The pre-taper is a 7-day process.

Statements of fact: All psychoactive medications metabolize through specific pathways. All psychoactive medications alter the Hypothalamic Pituitary-Adrenal Axis to some degree. To some extent, you can predict the duration before drug-adverse reactions begin with most psychoactive drugs; if the patient's P450 (CYP) enzymes have been screened. A poor metabolizer as well as an extensive metabolizer will eventually reach the same saturation point; the poor metabolizer much faster, of course. If one were to look at the basic structure of the human body, the chemical structure of psychiatric drugs, and include how psychiatric drugs are metabolized, how foods, vitamins, minerals, DNA, amino acids, hormones, glands, proteins, fatty acids and enzymes work, in relation to psychiatric drugs, you have The Road Back Science

The patient has been under some duress and stress before a diagnosis was given and the prescription was written. With this in mind the patients JNK gene would have been overly expressed for some duration. Balancing the JNK gene activation will lead to a normalization of the patient in time.

Drug targets for most disorders will be the purinergic system, the dynorphin opioid neuropeptide system, the cholinergic system (muscarinic and nicotinic systems), the melatonin and serotonin system, and the HPA axis. An

156

additional reason the supplements were selected to be used in this program; their natural action of helping to balance the same drug targets.

DNA and Prediction of Drug Adverse Reactions

The following charts detail the P450 enzymes used to metabolize the most common antidepressants, anti-psychotics, benzodiazepines and ADHD stimulant medications. An X in the row denotes that the medication utilizes that specific pathway. Below each chart, you will find other routes of metabolism if applicable.

These medications *inhibit* metabolism via listed CYP pathways.

Drug	P450 Enzyme Pathway				
Antidepressants	**1A2**	**2C19**	**2C9**	**2D6**	**3A**
* Adapin	X	X	X	X	
* Anafranil	X	X		X	X
*Apo-Amitriptyline	X	X	X	X	
*Apo- Clomipramine	X	X		X	
* Apo-Doxepin	X	X	X	X	
* Apo-Imipramine	X	X		X	
* Apo-Selegiline	X	X			
* Apo-Trimip		X	X	X	
* Celexa		X		X	
Cymbalta	X			X	
* Desyrel				X	
* Elavil	X	X		X	
* Eldepryl	X	X			
* Effexor				X	X
* Effexor XR				X	
Lexapro		X		X	

157

* Ludiomil				X	
* Luvox	X	X	X	X	X
* Norpramin				X	
* Novo-					
* Novo-	X	X			
*Novo-		X	X	X	
*Nu-		X	X	X	
* Pamelor				X	X
* Paxil	X	X	X	X	
* Paxil CR	X	X		X	
*PMS-				X	
* Prozac	X	X	X	X	X

Remeron	X			X	X
* Rhotrimine		X	X	X	
Sarafem	X	X	X	X	X
Serzone					X
Sinequan	X	X	X	X	
Strattera		X		X	
* Surmontil		X	X	X	
* Tofranil	X	X		X	X
* Triptil				X	
* Vivactil				X	
Trazodone				X	X
* Wellbutrin	X		X	X	X
* Wellbutrin SR				X	
* Zoloft	X	X	X	X	X
*Zonalon Topical	X	X	X	X	
* Zyban				X	

Marked medications (*) will also use other routes for metabolism:

158

Adapin – ABCB1-P-pg, UGT1A3, UGT1A4

Anafranil – UGT2B10, CYP3A4, UGT1A4, UGT1A4, UGT2B7, ABCB1-P-gp, CYP3A4

Apo-Amitriptyline – 3A4, UGT2B10, UGT1A4, SLC22A1- OCT1, ABCB1-P-gp, UGT2B7, CYP3A4, CYP2C8, CYP2D6

Apo-Clomipramine – UGT2B10, CYP3A4, UGT1A4,UGT2B7, UGT1A4, UGT1A3

Apo-Doxepin – ABCB1-P-gp, UGT1A3, UGT1A4

Apo-Imipramine – UGT2B10, ABCB1-P-gp, UGT1A4, CYP3A4, SLC22A2-OCT2, UGT1A3, UGT2B7, SLC22A1-OCT1, SLC22A3-OCT3, CYP3A4

Apo-Selegiline – CYP2B6, CYP2C8, CYP3A4, CYP2A6, MAO-B

Apo-Trimip – UGT1A4, CYP3A4, UGT2B10, ABCB1-P-gp

Celexa – ABCB1-P-gp, CYP3A4

Desyrel – CYP3A4, ABCB1-P-gp, P-pg Effexor – CYP3A4, ABCB1-P-gp, P-gp Effexor XR – CYP3A4, ABCB1-P-gp, P-gp

Elavil – UGT1A4, UGT1A3, P-gp

Eldepryl – CYP2B6, CYP2C8, CYP3A4, CYP2A6, MAO-B

Ludiomil – ABCB1-P-gp

Luvox – 2B6, P-gp, intestinal 3A, ABCB1-P-gp, CYP2B6, CYP3A4

Norpramin – SLCC22A1-OCT1, SLC22A2-OCT2, SLC22A3-OCT3, CYP3A4

Novo-Doxepin – ABCB1-P-gp, UGT1A3, UGT1A3, UGT1A4

Novo-Selegiline – CYP2B6, CYP2C8, CYP3A4, CYP2A6, MAO-B

Novo-Tripramine – UGT1A4, CYP3A4, UGT2B10, ABCB1-P-gp

Nu-Trimipramine – UGT1A4, CYP3A4, UGT2B10, ABCB1-P-gp

Pamelor – CYP3A4, ABCB1-P-gp, CYP2C8

Paxil – 2B6, P-gp, CYP3A4, CYP2B6, ABCB1-P-gp

Paxil CR – CYP3A4, CYP2B6,ABCR1-P-gp

PMS-Desipramine – SLC22A1-OCT1, SLC22A2-OCT2, SLC22A3-OCT3, CYP3A4

Prozac – 2B6, P-gp, ABCG2-BCRP, SLC22A3-OCT3, CYP3A4, SLC22A1-OCT1, ABCB1-P-gp

Rhotrimine – UGT1A4, CYP3A4, UGT2B10, ABCB1-P-gp Sarafem – 2B6, P-gp, ABCG2-BCRP, SLC22A3-OCT3, CYP3A4, SLC22A1-OCT1, ABCB1-P-gp

Serzone -- U

Sinequan – UBCB1-P-gp, UGT1A3, UGT1A4

Surmontil – UGT1A4, CYP3A4, UGT2B10, ABCB1-P-gp

Tofranil – UGT1A4, UGT1A3, P-gp, Triptil – ABCB1-P-gp

Vivactil – ABCB1-P-gp

Wellbutrin – 2E1, 2A6, 2B6, CYP2B6

Wellbutrin SR – CYP2B6

Zoloft – UGT2B7, UGT1A4, P-gp, 2B6, CYP2B6, MAO, CYP3A4, ABCB1-P-gp

Zonalon Topical Crème – ABCB1-P-gp, UGT1A3, UGT1A4

Zyban – CYP2B6

Drug	P450 Enzyme Pathway				
Anti-psychotics	**1A2**	**2C19**	**2C9**	**2D6**	**3A**
Abilify				X	X
* Apo-					
Perphenazine	X	X		X	
* Apo-					
Thioridazine	X			X	
* Chlorprom				X	
*Chlorpromanyl	X				
* Clozaril	X	X	X	X	X
* Geodon	X				X
* Haldol	X			X	
* Haldol					
Decanoate	X			X	
* Mellaril	X			X	X
Navane	X			X	
*Novo-Chlorpromazine	X				
* Novo-					
Ridazine	X				
* Orap	X			X	X
* Permitil	X			X	
* PMS-					
Perphenazine	X				
* Prolixin	X			X	
Prolixin					
Decanoate	X			X	
Prolixin					

Drug	P450 Enzyme Pathway				
Anti-psychotics	1A2	2C19	2C9	2D6	3A
Enanthate	X			X	
* Risperdal				X	X
* Seroquel				X	X
* Serentil				X	
* Sparine	X	X	X		
* Stelazine	X				
* Thorazine				X	
* Tindal					
* Trilafon	X	X		X	
* Zyprexa	X			X	
Other					
Cogentin				X	
* Lithium					

Marked medications (*) will also use other routes for metabolism:

Apo-Perphenazine – CYP3A4, CES1

Apo-Thioridazine – UGT1A4, ABCB1-P-gp, CYP3A4, CES1

Chlorprom – UGT1A4, UGT1A3, P-gp

Chlorpromanyl – UGT1A4, ABCB1-P-gp

Clozaril – FMO, UGT1A4, UGT1A3, ABCB1-P-gp, FMO3, ABCG2-BCRP

Geodon – Aldehyde oxidase substrate

Haldol – Glucuronidation, P-gp, UGT2B7, CYP3A4,

CYP3A5, UGT1A9, ABCB1-P-gp

Haldol Decanoate – UGT2B7, CYP3A4, CYP3A5, UGT1A9, ABCB1-P-gp

Mellaril – CYP3A4, CES1, P-gp

Novo-Chlorpromazine – UGT1A4, ABCB1-P-gp

Novo-Ridazine – UGT1A4, ABCB1-P-gp

Orap – ABCB1 – P-gp, CYP3A4, P-gp

PMS-Perphenazine – UGT1A4, ABCB1-P-gp

Prolixin – P-gp

Risperdal – P-gp, renal extraction, CYP3A4, ABCB1-P-gp, ABCG2-BCRP

Seroquel – Glucuronidation, P-gp, intestinal 3A, epoxide by quetiapine, CYP3A4, ABG2-BCRP, ABCB1-P-gp

Sparine – CYP3A4

Stelazine – UGT1A4, ABCB1-P-gp, P-gp Thorazine – UGT1A4, UGT1A3, P-gp Tindal – CYP2A6

Trilafon – CYP3A4, CES1

Zyprexa – Glucuronidation, FMO, UGT1A4

Drug	P450 Enzyme Pathway				
Benzodiazepine Anti-anxiety Sleep Medication Anticonvulsant	1A2	2C19	2C9	2D6	3A
Alprazolam		X			X
Ambien	X		X		X
* Apo-Chiordiazepoxide					
* Apo-Diazepam		X			
* Apo-Oxazepam					
* Apo-Temazepam					
* Apo-Triazo					
* Ativan					
* Barbita	X	X	X		
* BuSpar				X	X
* Carbatrol	X	X	X		
* Depakene			X		
Celontin		X			
* Depakote	X	X	X		X
* Diastat		X			
* Diazemuls		X			
* Diazepam Intensol		X			
* Dilantin		X			X

164

Drug	P450 Enzyme Pathway				
Benzodiazepine Anti-anxiety Sleep Medication Anticonsulsant	1A2	2C19	2C9	2D6	3A
* Dizac		X			
* Doral			X		
* Epitol	X	X	X		
* Felbatol		X			X
* Gen-Xene	X	X	X	X	
* Halcion					X
* Klonopin					X
* Lamecital					
* Librium					X
* Neurontin					
* Novo-Triolam					
* Nu-Carbamazepine	X	X	X		
* Nu-Loraz					
* Oxepam					
* Paxipam					
* PMS-Clonazepam					
* PMS-Diazepam		X			
* ProSom					
* Restoril					
* Rivotril					
* Serax					
* Solfoton	X	X	X		
Tegretol	X	X	X		
* Tranxene		X			
* Trileptal		X			X
* Valium		X			X
* Vivol		X			

165

		X			X
* Xanax		X			X
* Zonegran		X			

Drug	P450 Enzyme Pathway				
	1A2	**2C19**	**2C9**	**2D6**	**3A**
* Zopax		X			
* Zarontin					

Marked medications (*) will also use other routes for metabolism:

Alprazolam – Hepatic 3A, CYP3A5, CYP3A4
Apo-Chiordiazepoxide – CYP3A4
Apo-Diazepam – CYP3A4, CYP2B6, CYP3A5, UGT2B7
Apo-Oxazepam – UGT2B15, UGT2B7
Apo-Temazepam – UGT2B15, UGT2B7
Apo-Triazo – CYP3A4, CYP3A5
Ativan – UGT2B15, UGT2B7
Barbita – UGT2B15, UGT1A9, UGT1A6, CYP2E1, CYP3A4, UGT2B7, CES1, UGT1A1, CYP2C8, CYP2B6, CYP2A6, SULT2A1
BuSpar – Intestinal 3A, 3a4
Carbatrol – 3A4, CYP2C8, SLC22A5-OCT2N, UGT2B7, CES1, CYP2B6, ABCB7-ASAT, SULT1A1, ABCC2-MRP2, ABCG2- BCRP, SLCO1A2-DATP1A2
Depakene – CYP2B6, UGT1A6, CYP2A6, UGT2B15, UGT2B7, UGT1A9, ABCB1-P-gp
Depakote – UGT2B7, UGT1A6, UGT1A9, UGT2B15, UGT1A4, UGT1A3
Diastat – CYP3A4, CYP2B6, CYP3A5, UGT2B7

Diazemuls – CYP3A4, CYP2B6, CYP3A5, UGT287
Diazepam Intensol – CYP3A4, CYP2B6, CYP3A5, UGT2B7
Dilantin – UGT1A4, UGT1A6, UGT1A9, ABCB1-P-gp, CYP2C9, CYP2C8, UGT1A1, CYP3A5, UGT2B7, CYP3A4, CYP2B6, UGT2B15
Dizac – CYP3A4, CYP2B6, CYP3A5,UGT2B7
Doral – CYP3A4, CYP2C19, FMO, CYP2B6
Epitol – CYP2C8, SLC22A5-OCTN2, UGT2B7,CES1, CYP2B6, ABCB7-ASAT, SULT1A1, ABCC2- MRP2, ABCG2-BCRP, CYP1A2, CYP3A5
Felbatol – CYP2E1, CYP3A4
Gen-Xene – NAT2
Helicion – CYP3A4, CYP3A5
Klonopin – NAT2, CYP3A4
Lamictal – UGT1A3, UGT2B7, UGT1A4
Librium – CYP3A4
Luminal – UGT2B15
Neurontin – SLC22A4-OCTN1
Novo-Triolam – CYP3A4, CYP3A5
Nu-Carbamazepine – CYP2C8, SLC22A5-OCTN2, UGT2B7, CES1, CYP2B6, CYP3A4, ABCB7-ASAT, SULT1A1, ABCC2-MRP2, CYP3A5
Nu-Loraz – UGT2B15, UGT2B7
Oxepam – UGT2B15, UGT2B7
Paxipam – UGT2B7, UGT1A9, UGT2B15
PMS-Clonazepam – NAT2, CYP3A4
PMS-Diazepam – CYP3A4, CYP2B6, CYP3A5, UGT2B7
ProSom – CYP3A4
Restoril – UGT2B15, UGT2B7
Rivotril – NAT2, CYP3A4
Serax – UGT2B15, UGT2B7, UGT1A9
  Solfoton – UGT2B15, UGT1A9, UGT1A6, CYP2E1,

167

CYP3A4, UGT2B7, CEST1, UGT1A1, CYP2C8,
CYP2B6, CYP2A6, SULT2A1
Tegretol – 3A4, CYP2C8, SLC22A5-OCTN2, UGT2B7
Tranxene – CYP3A4, UGT2B7, UGT1A9, UGT2B15
Trileptal – CYP3A4, CYP3A5, UGT1A4
Valium – CYP2B6, UGT2B7, intestinal 3A, CYP3A4,
CYP3A5, Vivol – CYP3A4, CYP2B6, CYP3A5,
UGT2B7
Xanax – Hepatic 3A, CYP3A5, CYP3A4
Zonegran – NAT2, CYP3A4
Zopax – CYP3A4, CYP3A5
Zarontin – CYP3A4, CYP2E1

Drug	P450 Enzyme Pathway				
ADD/ADHD	1A2	2C19	2C9	2D6	3A
Adderall				X	
* Concerta				X	
Dextrostat				X	
* Medate		X		X	
* Methylin		X		X	
* Ritalin		X		X	
* Ritalin LA		X		X	
Strattera		X		X	
* Vyvanse	X			X	

Marked medications (*) will also use other routes for
metabolism:
Concerta – Glucuronidation, CES1A1. Medate –
CES1A1.
Methylin – CES1A1.
Ritalin – Glucuronidation, CES1A1. Ritalin – CES1A1.
Vyvanse – CYP3A4, MAO

How to Use Charts to Decide Sequence of Medication Reduction

If you have two or more medications sharing the same CYP pathway to metabolize, reduce the medication that uses the fewest pathways first.

Example: Ambien used concurrently with Luvox, Paxil, Prozac, Wellbutrin or Zoloft. Reduce the Ambien first.

If you were to reduce any of the antidepressants listed first, the Ambien would begin to clear the body faster and the patient would experience Ambien withdrawal without the current Ambien dosage being reduced. Ambien would be reduced by as much as 43% if the antidepressant were reduced first. (See Ambien product insert.)

The best approach is to always taper the anticonvulsant, antianxiety, benzodiazepine or sleep medication first and then tackle the antipsychotic and antidepressant.

If taking two antidepressants concurrently, or taking an antidepressant and an antipsychotic, selecting which one to reduce first would also follow the format outlined earlier in this section. The drug using fewer common CYP pathways should be reduced first.

If taking two antidepressants or one antidepressant and one antipsychotic, and the CYP pathways match, evaluate the current side effects, when each side effect started, when each medication was introduced, and determine from those side effects which taper schedule to follow and which drug to taper first.

From time to time, a person will also be taking a drug as an inducer of the CYP pathways.

Determine if this "inducer" was prescribed to help offset the inhibitor drug's effect or is the *inducer* drug prescribed for other health reasons not related.

You will generally find that those who are also taking the *inducer* medication will be suffering from a wide variety of adverse side effects. When reducing any medication attached to the same pathway as an inducer medication, reduce the normal taper speed by one-half for at least the first 2 months.

You may need to alternate reduction of the inducer drug and the inhibitor drug every other reduction in order to maintain a balance.

Other medications must be closely evaluated. Lipitor, as an example, is an inhibitor of the CYP 2C19, 2D6, and 3A, along with inhibiting the UGT1A3, UGT1A1, P-gp, and intestinal 3A.

Use drug product inserts to determine metabolism route or the Physicians' Desk Reference.

Example 1: If taking multiple medications and each medication uses the same metabolic route, each of the medications is competing for clearance. If one medication is reduced, the other medications will also be reduced or clear the body faster.

Decide which medication to taper off first based on:

• CYP charts

• Full evaluation of side effects

• When side effects started with which medication.

If patient has used Lexapro for two years and used Risperdal for 2 months and side effects increased dramatically once Risperdal was introduced, taper the Risperdal first.

Example 2: If multiple medications are being taken and all medications can metabolize through several routes, the impact will be lessened, and selecting which medication to taper first would not be pathway dependent.

Avoid all *supplements* that compete with the same pathways, and eliminate as much as possible all foods that compete with the medication by inducing or inhibiting the metabolism routes of the medications.

With the advancements of The Road Back Program, as described in this book, patients can now taper off antidepressants, antipsychotics and ADHD medications and stimulants simultaneously. Reduce the medications as slowly as possible, as close to 10% reduction as possible, and only increase the rate of reduction once the patient has shown tapering success at lower reductions.

Supplements, Herbs and Foods

Supplements, herbs or certain foods can have a direct impact on the success of the taper.

Datum: If a person smokes or drinks coffee before starting the pre- taper, do not suggest they quit. Cigarette smoke induces the CYP1A2, 2E1, 3A and UGT2B7. Nicotine inhibits UGT1A1, UGT1A4, UGT2A6, and UGT1A9. If taking Depakote and starting or stopping smoking, the impact on the medication will be dramatic.

If a patient starts to smoke or quits smoking while taking Cymbalta, the drug will be altered by as much as 15%. In theory, this should

171

apply as well to any other drugs sharing the same metabolism routes.

Coffee or caffeine inhibits the CYP1A2, 2E1 and the 3A. A high percentage of these medications metabolize through these pathways and caffeine usage will dramatically increase the medication, or if the person were to quit drinking caffeine, they would begin to go into withdrawal to some degree because the pathways will begin to metabolize the medication faster.

The times a person takes medication and when they drink two cups of coffee can have an impact as well. If the person drinks two cups of coffee every morning about one hour after their medication, and they change the time of the morning they drink the coffee, expect a slight to above average side effect from the medication.

The person's current daily routine should not be changed. If they were on a poor diet before starting this program, do not change their diet drastically. If they did not exercise before starting this program, do not advise them to do more than a casual walk.

Once off all medication for 45 days, a healthy diet can be implemented, an exercise program that matches their current physical condition can be started, the patient can stop smoking, etc.

A trace amount of an herb or supplement *will not* create an adverse reaction or alter the metabolism speed.

DNA Drug Reaction Testing and Taper Prediction

For the past several years, DNA drug reaction testing has been available to determine the patient's ability to metabolize medication through the CYP450 enzymes.

We have conducted over 200 drug reaction tests with the objective of determining how well drug-adverse reactions could be predicted, and if there were clinical use of this DNA data for tapering.

Prediction of a drug-adverse reaction: The individuals who were slow or poor metabolizers or hyper metabolizers experienced drug-adverse reactions faster than normal or intermediate metabolizers.

However, the normal or intermediate metabolizers still experienced adverse drug reactions, but after longer usage of the medication. *The metabolism type of the individual was not indicative of the severity of adverse reactions or duration.* Once the drug had saturated the CYP enzyme used for metabolism, all the individuals experienced the same side effect profile regardless of their metabolism speed noted from the DNA drug reaction test.

The test results from the DNA drug-reaction test did not lead to a worthwhile taper guide. It was postulated; if you were to induce the enzymes or inhibit an enzyme to match a specific test result and medication, you would be better able to adjust the metabolism and avoid withdrawal, or predict the withdrawal sequence. Again, this did not assist in tapering or eliminating withdrawal side effects in the slightest. This seems to parallel the results using an inducer drug to counteract the inhibition of the main drug.

If a DNA drug-reaction test has any use to a physician, it would be for predicting the dosage of the medication Coumadin. The initial prescription could be limited to a narrow band, and the correct therapeutic dosage would be found in a few weeks, instead of several months.

Nutritional DNA Test

Nutritional DNA testing provided this program substantial information to work with. We tested the ability of over 100 subjects to metabolize B vitamins, folate, calcium, Omega 3, phase II liver detox genes, Interleukin-6, and an assortment of other genetic differences that ultimately determine overall health and physical well-being.

The Road Back Program and all suggested nutritionals used for medication tapering address the most common genetic variations of the population at large. Though DNA science is not precise at this date, enough evidence is available to formulate part of a program to address the highest percentage of the population.

Hypothalamic-Pituitary-Adrenal Axis (HPA)

Psychoactive medications play havoc with the HPA. While benzodiazepines usually help with anxiety for a certain time period, the feedback loop sending incorrect data will eventually cause cortisol levels to increase, and the result will be increased anxiety in the morning and mid-afternoon. Insomnia will usually follow the cortisol level increase. Other psychoactive medications have their own unique side effect profile and ultimate effect upon the HPA.

First year medical school textbooks describe the hypothalamus as: "Hypothalamus/ homeostasis or maintaining the body's status quo." As an example, blood pressure, body temperature, fluid, the electrolyte balance and body weight are held in a precise value labeled the "set-point." The body's set-point may change over time, but from day to day, the set-point will remain nearly fixed. With the HPA receiving continual input about the state of the body and the ability of the HPA to initiate changes, as anything might sporadically fall out of balance, it is vital for the HPA to have at hand all necessary nutrients to assist with the compensation.

When the HPA is out of balance, you will have a problem with insulin, stress, anxiety, weight gain, thyroid problems, fatigue, unbalanced sexual hormones and countless other body difficulties.

The hormone, ACTH, will eventually become out of balance, as will the other hormones and adrenals.

Psychoactive medication directly alters specific areas within the HPA. Examine any patient using psychoactive medication for more than three months and you will probably find a problem with hormones, thyroid, adrenals, cortisol and immune system or other areas within the HPA.

However, it will be equally important to move beyond the normal view of the HPA. Psychoactive medication side effects are quite varied and diverse. This is not to rehash data from medical school, but to tie in the knowledge gained in the educational process with psychoactive medication.

Some fibers from the optic nerve go directly to a small nucleus within the hypothalamus (suprachiasmatic nucleus). This nucleus regulates circadian rhythms, and couples the rhythms to the light/dark cycles.

The nucleus of the solitary tract will collect sensory data from the vagus and relay the data to the hypothalamus. This data will include blood pressure and gut enlargement.

The reticular formation receives a vast supply of inputs from the spinal cord and relays that data to the hypothalamus. Part of that data will be skin temperature.

Nuclei, circumventricular organs, are unique in their own right as they lack a blood-brain barrier. They monitor substances in the blood and have the ability to monitor substances normally shielded by the neural tissue. Here you will find regulation of fluid and electrolyte balance, by controlling thirst, sodium excretion, blood volume regulation and vasopressin secretion. Include in this the area postrema, and you have the detection of blood toxins and the vomit-inducing center. The OVLT and area postrema project to the hypothalamus.

The limbic and olfactory systems project to the hypothalamus. Psychoactive medication side effects, such as eating problems and reproduction difficulty, will probably be traced to this area.

Ionic balance and temperature will be subject to the hypothalamus via the receptors, thermoreceptor and osmorecepter.

When the hypothalamus is aware of a problem, it will assert repair mechanisms. Neural signals to the autonomic system will attempt to regulate heart rate, vasoconstriction, digestion, sweating etc, and the endocrine signals to and or through the pituitary.

The pituitary side effects will include one or all six hormones, to include ACTH and the thyroid-stimulating hormone (TSH). The repair output attempt, and the psychoactive medication side effect profile, seem to run near a 50 percent occurrence. Furthermore, you can directly trace psychoactive medication side effects to the autonomic nervous system in both the sympathetic and

176

parasympathetic systems.

The hypothalamus can alter blood pressure; control every endocrine gland in the body, body temperature, adrenal levels via ACTH, and metabolism.

The repetition of HPA information in this chapter has been intentional. Do not be surprised to find a male patient with extremely high estrogen levels, a female with high testosterone or any other problems that can be associated within the HPA axis.

Taper the medication first, wait 45 days after the last dosage of the medication, reevaluate the patient, and then gradually bring all parts of the HPA back into balance. The nutritionals used with The Road Back Program were developed to help the body overcome this imbalance *gradually*. Gradually is italicized because this is where most problems occur with psychoactive drug-taper programs. Either they do not address the HPA or the program is really a detoxification or heavy metal chelating program.

The Road Back Program utilizes specific nutritionals to address the drug side effects and to begin the process of balancing the HPA. Specifics on each nutritional, what each nutritional is addressing within the HPA or the body in relation to psychoactive medications, can be found in The Road Back Program patent when published by the U.S. Patent Office.

Immune System

The immune system and the HPA are in constant communication and actions within one system will induce response in the other. The supplements used in this program are designed to also influence the immune response.

Reducing oxidative stress has been shown to balance Interleukin-2 (IL-2) as well as Interleukin-6. If you were to test your bipolar patients IL-2 levels, you will find they will be too high during the manic phase and IL-6 levels will have shot up high during the depressive phase. A schizophrenic will have either too high or too low IL-2 levels and will usually exhibit high IL-6 levels constantly.

The JNK supplement will reduce oxidative stress and lower IL-2 levels as well as IL-6 levels. The specific cascading effect is; JNK gene over expression leads to increase of Interleukin-2 levels which create an imbalance of Th1 and Th2. CD4 will usually show dysfunction after prolonged Th1 and Th2 alteration.

Titrating Medication

The Road Back has tried titrating medication gradually without the use of nutritionals with limited success. About 50% of the people could taper off their medication without using these nutritionals but they still suffered extreme withdrawal side effects.

Using a gradual titration combined with a basic detoxification approach had lower than 50% success.

The normal supplements used to remove heavy metal or for a liver detox produced undesirable results.

A gradual titration with the use of the suggested nutritionals gives our standard successful results.

The Key to a Successful Taper With The Road Back Program

Following the pre-taper exactly as described is critical. The pre-taper is the make or break point for every successful taper.

Most problems occur when:

- The pre-taper is done too quickly.

- Patient does not stop increasing a nutritional once a positive change occurs.

- Patient changes the time of day they take medication.

- Patient changes the time of day they take nutritionals.

- Medication is reduced too quickly.

- A new medication is prescribed in addition to existing medication.

- Patient is switched to a new medication.

- Doctor has patient use additional supplements or vitamins not in this program.

- Patient begins taking other supplements.

- Patient makes a major change to their daily routine.

- Patient skips days of taking medication.

Titrating Psychoactive Medication:

Have the patient compound his/her medication whenever possible. An exact reduction of the medication each week provides prediction, no guessing, and the highest chance of success.

In the early days of psychoactive drugs, psychiatry did not titrate psychoactive drugs up slowly on patients and the results were catastrophic. Many drugs, other than psychoactive drugs, must be titrated up as well as down before complete discontinuing.

There seems to be a medical community consensus that psychoactive drugs can be reduced quickly, or patients can abruptly be taken off one psychoactive drug and prescribed another psychoactive drug without an adverse consequence. This is not the case. Even switching a patient from a tablet form of a psychoactive drug to the liquid form of the same psychoactive drug can cause extreme adverse drug reactions.

Dr. Donald E. McAlpine, psychiatrists at the Mayo Clinic states: *"It's important to taper off slowly, extending the taper over several weeks under your physician's direction. When you stop too quickly, you may experience so-called discontinuation symptoms, which can masquerade as relapse."*

The discontinuation process and side effects therein can be confusing to both the patient and physician. Which side effect is coming from the medication, or is it a return of the original symptom?

With a full pre-taper completed before reducing the medication, rest assured the side effect starting during the taper is due to one of the following:

The patient changed something.

The reduction of the medication is too large.

A change made by the patient can be the most difficult to find. It might be something the patient does not feel is a change.

Years ago, I had a person nearly halfway off Paxil. This person experienced no withdrawal side effects tapering the Paxil to that point. When trying to taper off Paxil in the past, the individual had extreme withdrawal side effects after the first reduction attempt and would then need to return to a full dosage.

With no valid explanation, this person began to suffer withdrawal side effect symptoms similar to those earlier. Two weeks passed and I could not find anything the person had changed. Finally, it was mentioned to me by the individual he or she had started an all-protein diet, began the diet 3 days before the side effects started.

For this person doing this diet was not a change. He or she would go on this all-protein diet every six months. I give you this example to point out that the change a patient makes may not be so obvious. You may need to dig.

If a patient is keeping a complete Daily Journal these changes can be spotted more quickly and trouble tapering can be avoided.

Use the Suggested Supplements

If you want the standard results with The Road Back Program, use the exact supplements suggested. Read through the chapter, "Nutritionals" Used on The Road Back Program for a list of all supplements, basic description of each and where they are available. Most, if not all of the manufacturers of these supplements offer a healthcare provider distributor program, if you wish to carry them in your practice.

Bailey, L.B., Gregory, J.F., (1999). *"Polymorphisms of methylenetetrahydrofolate reductase and other enzymes: metabolic significance, risks and impact on folate requirement."* J Nutr 129(5): 919-22.

Bailey, L.B., Gregory, J.F., (1999). *"Folate metabolism and requirements."* J Nutr 129(4): 779-82. Basile, V.S., Masellis, M., Potkin, S.G., Kennedy, J.L., Pharmacogenomics in schizophrenia: the quest for individualized therapy. Hum Mol Genet. 2002 Oct 1;11(20):2517-30

Blaisdell, J., Mohrenweiser, H., Jackson, Ferguson, J., Coulter, S., Chanas, S., Chanas, B., Xi, T., Ghanayem, B., Goldstein, J.A. Identification and functional characterization of new potentially defective alleles of human CYP2C19. Pharmacogenetics. 2002 Dec;12(9):703-11.

Bosron, W.F., Ting-Kai, L., (1986). "Genetic polymorphism of human liver alcohol and aldehyde dehydrogenases, and their relationship to alcohol metabolism and alcoholism." Hepatology 6(3): 502 – 510.

Bradford, L.D., CYP2D6 allele frequency in European Caucasians, Asians, Africans and their descendants. Pharmacogenomics. 2002 Mar;3 (2):229-43.

Brockmoller, J., et.al. Pharmacogenetic diagnosis of cytochrome P450 polymorphisms in clinical drug development and in drug treatment. Pharmacogenetics. 2000:1:125-51.

Budziszewska B, Szymanska M, Leskiewicz M, Basta-Kaim A, Jaworska-Feil L, Kubera M, Jantas D, Lason W. The decrease in JNK- and p38-MAP kinase activity is accompanied by the enhancement of PP2A phosphate level in the brain of prenatally stressed rats. J Physiol Pharmacol. 2010 Apr;61(2):207-15.

C. Mastronardi, G J Paz-Filho, E Valdez, J Maestre-Mesa, J Licinio, and M-L Wong. Long-term body weight outcomes of antidepressant environment interactions. Mol Psychiatry 2011 March, (16)3:265-272

Carter CJ. Multiple genes and factors associated with bipolar disorder converge on growth factor and stress activated kinase pathways controlling translation initiation: implications for oligodendrocyte viability. Neurochem Int. 2007 Feb;50(3):461-90. Epub 2007 Jan 18. Review.

Ceriello, A., Giugliano, D., Quatraro, A., Lefebvre, P.J., Anti-oxidants show an anti-hypertensive effect in diabetic and hypertensive subjects. Clin Sci 1991;81:739-42.

Chang, T.K., et al. Enhanced cyclophosphamide and ifosfamide activation in primary human hepatocyte cultures: response to cytochrome P-450 inducers and autoinduction by oxazaphosphorines. Cancer Res 1997; 57(10):1946-54.

Chango, A., Boisson, F., et al. (2000). *"The effect of 677C-->T and 1298A-->C mutations on plasma homocysteine and 5,10-methylenetetrahydrofolate reductase activity in healthy subjects."* Br J Nutr 83(6): 593-6.

Charradi K, Sebai H, Elkahoui S, Ben Hassine F, Limam F, Aouani E. Grape Seed Extract Alleviates High-Fat Diet-Induced Obesity and Heart Dysfunction by Preventing Cardiac Siderosis. Cardiovasc Toxicol. 2011 Jan 14.

Cheng, T., Zhu, Z., et al. (2001). *"Effects of multinutrient supplementation on antioxidant defense systems in healthy human beings."* J Nutr Biochem 12(7): 388-395.

Chida, M., Yokoi, T., Fukui, T., Kinoshita, M., Yokota, J., Kamataki, T., Detection of three genetic polymorphisms in the 5'-flanking region and intron 1 of human CYP1A2 in the Japanese population. Jpn J Cancer Res. 1999 Sep;90(9):899-902

Chistyakov, D. A., Savost'anov, et al. (2001). *"Polymorphisms in the Mn-SOD and EC- SOD genes and their relationship to diabetic neuropathy in type 1 diabetes mellitus."* BMC Med Genet 2(1): 4.

Cosma, G., Crofts, F., et al. (1993). *"Relationship between genotype and function of the human CYP1A1 gene."* J Toxicol Environ Health 40(2-3): 309-16.

Cozza, K.L., Armstrong, S.C., Oesterheld, J.R., Drug Interaction principles for Medical Practice. American Psychiatric Publishing Inc. (2003)

Chuang DM. Neuroprotective and neurotrophic actions of the mood stabilizer lithium: can it be used to treat neurodegenerative diseases? Crit Rev Neurobiol. 2004;16(1-2):83-90. Review.

Das J et al. Acetaminophen induced acute liver failure via oxidative stress and JNK activation: protective role of taurine by the suppression of cytochrome P450 2E1. Free Radic Res. 2010; 44(3): 340-55.

Gao N, Budhraja A, Cheng S, Yao H, Zhang Z, Shi X. Induction of apoptosis in human leukemia cells by grape seed extract occurs via activation of c-Jun NH2-terminal kinase. Clin Cancer Res. 2009 Jan 1;15(1):140-9.

Ho, P.C., et al. Influence of CYP2C9 genotypes on the formation of a hepatotoxic metabolite of valproic acid in human liver microsomes. Pharmacogenomics J 2003; 3(6):335-42.

Jeong SW, Kim LS, Hur D, Bae W Y, Kim JR, Lee JH. Gentamicin-induced spiral ganglion cell death: apoptosis mediated by ROS and the JNK signaling pathway. Acta Otolaryngol. 2010 Jun;130(6):670-8.

Krause KH, Bonjpour JP, Berlit P, Kynast G, Schmidt-Gayk H, Schellenberg B. Effect of long-term treatment with antiepileptic drugs on vitamin status. Drug Nutr Interact. 1988;5(4):317-43.

Krause KH, Bonjour JP, Berlit P, Kochen W. Biotin status of epilitics. Ann NY Acad of Sci. 1985;447-297-313.

Krause KH, Bonjour JP, Berlit P, Kochen W. Excretion of organic acids associated with biotin deficiency in chronic anticonvulsant therapy. Int J Vitam Nutr Res. 1984;54(2-3);217-22.

Lam, Y.W.F., Gaedigk, A., Ereshefsy, L., et al: CYP2D6 inhibition by selective serotonin reuptake inhibitors: analysis of achievable steady-state plasma concentrations and the effect of ultrarapid metabolism at CYP2D6. Pharmacotherapy 2002;22:1001-1006.

Lichtenstein AH, Appel LJ, Brands M et al. Diet and lifestyle recommendations revision 2006: a scientific statement from the American Heart Association Nutrition Committee. Circulation, 2006 ; 114: 82-96.

Lin CL, Lin JK. Epigallocatechin gallate (EGCG) attenuates high glucose-induced insulin signaling blockade in human hepG2 hepatoma cells. Mol Nutr Food Res. 2008; 52(8): 930-9.

Liu H, Xiao Y, Xiong C, Wei A, Ruan J. Apoptosis induced by a new flavonoid in human hepatoma HepG2 cells involves   reactive oxygen species-mediated   mitochondrial dysfunction and MAPK activation. Eur J Pharmacol. 2011 Jan 15.

Madhyastha R, Madhyastha H, Nakajima Y, Omura S, Maruyama M. Curcumin Facilitates Fibrinolysis and Cellular Migration during Wound Healing by Modulating Urokinase Plasminogen Activator Expression. Pathophysiol Haemost Thromb. 2010 Nov 12

Maheshwari A, Misro MM, Aggarwal A, Sharma RK, Nandan D. N-Acetyl-L-cysteine counteracts oxidative stress and prevents H(2) O(2) induced germ cell apoptosis through down-regulation of caspase-9 and JNK/c-Jun. Mol Reprod Dev. 2010 Dec 22. doi: 10.1002/ mrd.21268.

Mock DM, Dvken ME, Biotin catabolism is accelerated in adults receiving long-term therapy with anticonvulsants. Department of Pediatrics, University of Arkansas for medical Sciences, Arkansas Children's Hospital, Little Rock, Rock. Neurology 1997 Nov:49(5):144-7

Moon et al. Inhibitory effect of (-)-epigallocatechin-3-gallate on lipid accumulation of 3T3-L1 cells. Obesity (Silver Spring). 2007; 15(11): 2571-82.

Pan J, Xiao Q, Sheng CY, Hong Z, Yang HQ, Wang G, Ding JQ, Chen SD. Blockade of the translocation and activation of c-Jun N-terminal kinase 3 (JNK3) attenuates dopaminergic neuronal damage in mouse model of Parkinson's disease. Neurochem Int. 2009 Jun;54(7):418-25. Epub 2009 Jan 29.

Romier-Crouzet B, Van De Walle J, During A, Joly A, Rousseau C, Henry O, Larondelle Y, Schneider YJ. Inhibition of inflammatory mediators by polyphenolic plant extracts in human intestinal Caco-2 cells. Food Chem Toxicol. 2009 Jun;47(6):1221-30. Epub 2009 Feb 20.

Said HM, Redha R, Nylander W. Biotin transport in the human intestine: Inhibition by anticonvulsant drugs. Dept. of pediatric Gastroenterology, Vanderbilt University School of medicine, Nashville, TN. Am J. Clin Nutr, 1989 Jan;49(1):127-31.

Spiliotaki M, Salpeas V, Malitas P, Alevizos V, Moutsatsou P. Altered glucocorticoid receptor signaling cascade in lymphocytes of bipolar disorder patients. Psychoneuroendocrinology. 2006 Jul;31(6):748-60. Epub 2006 Apr 18.

Stornetta RL, Zhu JJ. Ras and Rap Signaling in Synaptic Plasticity and Mental Disorders. Neuroscientist. 2010 Apr 29.

Tian H, Zhang G, Li H, Zhang Q. Antioxidant NAC and AMPA/K A receptor antagonist DNQX inhibited JNK3 activation following global ischemia in rat hippocampus. Neurosci Res. 2003 Jun;46(2):191-7.

Wu H et al. JNK-dependent NFATc1 pathway positively regulates IL-13 gene expression induced by (-)-epigallocatechin-3-gallate in human basophilic KU812 cells. Free Radic Biol Med. 2009; 47(7): 1028-38.

Wu N et al. Taurine prevents free fatty acid-induced hepatic insulin resistance in association with inhiditing JNK1 activation and improving insulin signaling in vitro. Diabetes Res Clin Pract. 2010 ; 90(3): 288-90.

Xie N, Wang C, Lin Y, Li H, Chen L, Zhang T, Sun Y, Zhang Y, Yin D, Chi Z. The role of p38 MAPK in valproic acid induced microglia apoptosis. Neurosci Lett. 2010 Sep 20 ;482(1):51-6. Epub 2010 Jul 16.

Xu Y, Hou XY, Liu Y, Zong Y Y. Different protection of K252a and N-acetyl-L-cysteine against amyloid-beta peptide-induced cortical neuron apoptosis involving inhibition of MLK3-MKK7-JNK3 signal cascades. J Neurosci Res. 2009 Mar;87(4):918-27.

Yaniv SP, Lucki A, Klein E, Ben-Shachar D. Dexamethasone enhances the norepinephrine-induced ERK/MAPK intracellular pathway possibly via dysregulation of the alpha2-adrenergic receptor: implications for antidepressant drug mechanism of action. Eur J Cell Biol. 2010 Sep;89(9):712-22.

Zhang F, Lau SS, Monks TJ. The Cytoprotective Effect of N-acetyl-L-cysteine against ROS-induced Cytotoxicity is Independent of its Ability to Enhance Glutathione Synthesis. Toxicol Sci. 2010 Dec 6.

Made in the USA
Charleston, SC
03 November 2013